CONTRASTS IN HEALTH STATUS

VOLUME 2

A Strategy for Evaluating Health Services

DAVID M. KESSNER, *Project Director*
CAROLYN E. KALK, *Research Coordinator*
Health Services Research Study

INSTITUTE OF MEDICINE
NATIONAL ACADEMY OF SCIENCES

Washington, D.C. 1973

NOTICE: This study was undertaken under the aegis of the Institute of Medicine of the National Academy of Sciences. The Institute considers the problem discussed in this report to be of national significance. It also feels the resources of the Institute were particularly suited to conduct the study.

Persons were selected for their individual scholarly competence and judgment to form the Health Services Research Panel and conduct this study.

This report has been reviewed by a review committee of the Institute and by the Institute's Council. It has not been submitted for approval to the full memberships of the Institute or Academy, nor to the Council of the Academy. Responsibility for all aspects of this report therefore rests with the study group.

The Board on Medicine of the National Academy of Sciences was restructured as the Institute of Medicine during the summer of 1970.

Available from:

Printing and Publishing Office, National Academy of Sciences
2101 Constitution Avenue, Washington, D.C. 20418

Library of Congress Cataloging in Publication Data

Institute of Medicine. Panel on Health Services Research.
    A strategy for evaluating health services.

    (Contrasts in health status series, v. 2)
    Includes bibliographical references.
    1. Medical care—United States. I. Kessner, David M., ed. II. Kalk, Carolyn E., ed.
III. Title. IV. Series.
RA395.A3I55   362.1   73-3494
ISBN 0-309-02104-9

Printed in the United States of America

Acknowledgments

Acknowledgments are due many persons for the time and energy they spent organizing and executing this study. Without their perseverance this report would not have been possible.

Joseph G. Giacalone participated in the development of criteria for selecting tracer conditions and in the development of the epidemiologic reviews. The background research and collation of the literature for the tracer conditions was carried out by the following individuals: Diane I. McEldowney (middle ear infection and associated hearing loss and hypertension), Joyce L. Smith (visual disorders), Carol A. Rothman (iron-deficiency anemia), Carol B. Pinson (urinary tract infections), and Claire Taylor (carcinoma of the cervix). Science writer James Singer was instrumental in preparing the final draft of the study.

Barbara B. Smith, who provided the staff with the administrative support essential to completing this project, is gratefully acknowledged. Karen K. Porter deserves special mention for her meticulous preparation and proofreading of the final document.

In addition to the principal consultants and the staff members, many other colleagues have offered valuable suggestions and have given freely of their time. I wish to express my appreciation to all of these individuals for their continuing interest and support. Nevertheless, the responsibility for insufficiencies or inaccuracies in the design and execution of this program rests solely with the Panel on Health Services Research and its primary staff.

DAVID M. KESSNER, *Project Director*
Health Services Research Study

iv

Cervical Cancer

Hervy E. Averette   Isadore D. Rotkin   Abraham Lilienfeld
John J. Mikuta

Essential Hypertension

Charles du V Florey   Herbert G. Langford   Jeremiah Stamler
Edward D. Fries

Urinary Tract Infections

Edward H. Kass   William R. McCabe   Marvin Turck

Family Practitioners

Robert A. Babineau   Charles S. Burger   Philip G. Sanfacon
Bradley E. Brownlow   Fitzhugh Mayo   Randall Silver
James A. Burdette

Management and Systems Analysis

David C. Dellinger   Louis R. Pondy   Lewis A. Miller

Medical Care Evaluation

Eliot Friedson   Beverly C. Payne   John W. Williamson
Charles A. Metzner

Medical Economics

Sylvester E. Berki   Paul J. Feldstein   Michael Grossman

Sampling and Design

Irene Hess

SPONSORS

Major support for this study was provided by the Carnegie Corporation of New York. The work was also supported by the Fannie E. Ripple Foundation; Association for the Aid of Crippled Children; John Hancock Life Insurance Company; Office of Health Evaluation, Deputy Assistant Secretary, Evaluation and Monitoring, Department of Health, Education, and Welfare (Contract No. HEW-OS-70-130); and Office of Planning, Research, and Evaluation, Office of Economic Opportunity (Contract No. BIC-5243).

Contents

ACKNOWLEDGMENTS   iii

FOREWORD   ix
  John R. Hogness

PREFACE   xiii

CONCLUSIONS   1

RECOMMENDATIONS   3
  Information Needs for Health Evaluation;
  Further Development of the Tracer Methodology

SUMMARY   6
  Criteria for Tracers; Selected Tracers; Evaluation and Change

CHAPTER ONE
DEVELOPMENT OF THE TRACER METHOD   11
  The State of the Art; Criteria for Evaluating Candidate Tracers; Selection of
  a Set of Tracers; Applying Tracer Methodology: An Example; Costs and
  Manpower Requirements; References

CHAPTER TWO
MIDDLE EAR INFECTION AND ASSOCIATED
HEARING LOSS   29
  Summary; A Minimal-Care Plan for Middle Ear Infections in Children;
  Clinical Aspects; Epidemiology; Functional Impact; References; Bibliography

CHAPTER THREE
VISUAL DISORDERS   67
  Summary; A Plan for Vision Screening in Children 4–11 Years of Age;
  Epidemiology; Functional Impact; References; Bibliography

CHAPTER FOUR

IRON-DEFICIENCY ANEMIA   96

Summary; A Minimal-Care Plan for Anemia in Children (to Age 5);
Pathogenesis; Methodological Considerations; Epidemiology; Functional
Impact; References; Bibliography

CHAPTER FIVE

ESSENTIAL HYPERTENSION   119

Summary; A Minimal-Care Plan for Hypertension; Epidemiology;
Functional Impact; References; Bibliography

CHAPTER SIX

URINARY TRACT INFECTIONS   162

Summary; A Minimal-Care Plan for Significant Bacteriuria; Clinical
Aspects; Methodological Considerations; Epidemiology; Functional Impact;
References; Bibliography

CHAPTER SEVEN

CERVICAL CANCER   192

Summary; A Minimal-Care Plan for Carcinoma of the Cervix; Clinical
Aspects; Epidemiology; Functional Impact; References; Bibliography

Foreword

Beginning, perhaps, with Sir William Petty in the late seventeenth century, the annals of public health have been sprinkled with proposals to evaluate the costs, benefits, and efficacy of health care.

Sir William—called one of the earliest advocates of cost-benefit analysis by Harvard economist Rashi Fein—proposed the Crown undertake economic analyses of medical services. He argued that by spending money the government would improve care and diminish the impact of the plague, thereby saving lives. Saving lives, he reasoned, would increase productivity and, in the end, save the government money.

We have seen in our lifetime, and particularly since the mid-1950s, an increased effort to evaluate health services. We are no longer threatened by the plague, but we are faced nonetheless with acute health delivery problems. We know from the data we see, and suspect from our personal experiences, that many of these accompany the issues of health care quality and the degree to which increased expenditures can lead to better health. These issues are not new. What is new, however, is increasing public participation in the debate—and, as a result of the debate, increasing public involvement in the organization of health delivery. Even the most cursory glance at the proposed health legislation in Congress confirms that changes, perhaps sweeping changes, are in the offing. The old structures and conventions of health care delivery are constantly questioned, attacked, and confronted by proposals to overhaul our health system.

Yet, while many of the pressures for change center on the issue of

quality, there is a wide technological gulf between the need and de-
sire to assure quality of care on the one side, and the ability to do so
on the other. Much of the proposed legislation assumes that we either
have ready methods of quality assessment or can rapidly put together
the technology, manpower, and data base needed for evaluation on a
national scale.

This, unfortunately, is not the case.

Health care evaluation is still a new and rudimentary discipline.
Many existing proposals for evaluation are cumbersome and would be
costly to implement.

In July 1969 the Board on Medicine of the National Academy of
Sciences undertook a program to evaluate health service delivery.
Called "Contrasts in Health Status," the program was designed to:

● Analyze differences in health status among different groups of
people in our population

● Relate differences in health status to social, economic, medical
care, and behavioral characteristics

● Compare the effect of various arrangements for the delivery of
services on selected groups of people

Together, the objectives touch on significant public issues in health
policy. They reach to the core of the evaluation process, identifying
and isolating the kinds of data policy makers need to reshape existing
programs, initiate new programs, and allocate resources. In addition,
they require the development of evaluative tools to assist the public
need for quality assessment, assurance, and achievement.

In developing a method for assessing health care status, the study
focused on the premise that specific health problems could provide a
mechanism for viewing health status and care, and a strategy for scien-
tifically analyzing health systems. In effect, a set of problems could
become natural "tracers" that allow an investigator or evaluator to
examine selected parts or the entire matrix of a health system. Data
gathered by tracer analysis, moreover, could be fed back into the
health delivery system, providing a base for constantly upgrading the
quality and organization of care.

A limited test of the tracer method, reported in Volume III of this
study, indicates that the method holds promise for evaluating ambulatory care. It now needs to be tested, as a second step, in more and
diverse health delivery organizations and systems. Many settings are
appropriate for further testing—neighborhood health centers, new

health maintenance organizations, and university-based outpatient departments come to mind readily.

We should not delay testing; evaluation is too critical to shaping the health systems of the future to wait for a perfect method, one suitable to every delivery system, to be developed. The methods we have now should be tested in conjunction with one another, and their respective limitations, costs, and usefulness compared carefully. That is work we must not delay if we are to meet our responsibilities to the health needs of the nation.

Funding for the study came from many sources; the major contribution was provided by the Carnegie Corporation of New York. The Institute is indebted to each of these sources, and particularly to the Carnegie Corporation for its foresight and unstinting support.

JOHN R. HOGNESS, *President*
Institute of Medicine
National Academy of Sciences

Preface

This volume reports the development of the tracer methodology for evaluating ambulatory health services. The tasks undertaken to meet this objective include:

- Establishment of criteria for selecting tracers
- Selection of a set of tracers for evaluating various aspects of delivery of ambulatory medical services in a population cross section
- Development of minimal medical care treatment criteria for each health problem selected as a tracer
- Development of a comprehensive description of the epidemiology and a summary of the functional impact of each tracer

These tasks are discussed in the body of this volume. In sum, they form a strategy for evaluating health delivery systems. The frequency rates of tracer conditions gauge the health status of a population; the ratio of treated to untreated cases measures the proficiency of the delivery system in reaching its community; the processes of diagnosis and treatment, when compared to a set of criteria, reflect the quality of medical practice; and the outcome of the treatment highlights the composite social and medical environment to which the patient is exposed.

This volume also examines application of the tracer method in evaluating a hypothetical health delivery system. Some of this material appeared previously, in a slightly different form, in *Development of Methodology for Evaluation of Neighborhood Health Centers,* funded under contract number HEW-OS-70-130 by the U.S. Department of Health, Education, and Welfare. Volume I of *Contrasts in Health Status* extended the use of the tracer concept to infant mortality; Volume III of the study reports findings of field tests in ambulatory delivery systems of the set of tracers described in this volume.

SAMUEL M. NABRIT, *Chairman*
Panel on Health Services Research
Institute of Medicine

A Strategy for Evaluating Health Services

Conclusions

If effective and efficient methods of evaluating health services are to be developed, not only must systems for collecting basic data be considered, several key requirements for implementing any evaluative system must be addressed. These requirements include:

● Phasing—Any national health evaluation system will need to be rationally phased into implementation, requiring perhaps a decade for full implementation. It will not be possible to evaluate all health delivery systems or components immediately.

● Manpower—Skilled manpower is crucial to implementing health care evaluation. The implications for sophisticated manpower at the national or regional level to direct health system evaluations point to a critical shortage of skills and training programs.

● Methods—Development of additional techniques for health care evaluation is needed. To date no single technique or combination of techniques adequately and efficiently evaluates the entire range of health care services and responsibilities.

● Costs—Projected costs of health system evaluation programs must be carefully analyzed. The nation can ill afford an evaluation system that dramatically increases the costs of health services. The potential of any evaluation method for reducing the costs of health care must be carefully explored.

The tracer methodology provides a manageable approach to dealing with many intricate problems in health evaluation. By expanding

1

the number of tracers—and combining the tracer technique with a structured and easily retrievable data base—a major step can be taken toward the development of a functional approach to health care evaluation. However, the quality and availability of community census data will need to be improved, and alternative methods for retrieving the data will need to be developed. The collection of community data will have to be better geared to the needs and problems of program administrators. Also health systems will need to develop mechanisms for translating evaluation results into actual changes in the delivery of health services.

Two factors are central to any strategy to evaluate ambulatory health services: medical records kept by health care providers and acceptance of minimal criteria for treating specific types of illnesses.

1. Records—Regardless of the method of evaluation used, it is impossible to tell what services were provided to the patient and by whom without a competently structured record system. As more services come to be furnished by nonphysicians, the need for structured records becomes more acute. Each provider, whether physician, nurse, paramedic, or social worker, must be able to determine easily which services were given by other providers and which services are needed in follow-up.

2. Criteria—Without minimal care criteria, it is impossible to judge if appropriate treatment was given. Several cautions, however, must be emphasized in establishing treatment criteria, or protocols, for the morbidity conditions used as tracers. Of utmost importance is the fact that no single standard can cope with the day-to-day variations faced by the practicing physician. The criteria cannot be assumed to be a rigid formula applicable to each individual patient. They can, and should, however, be applicable to the aggregate of patients. Further, the criteria must take into account not only the best thinking in the medical community regarding treatment of a specific condition, but also the practical constraints of the particular practice to be evaluated. These include availability of ancillary facilities and consultants, physician—population ratios and patient load, and the health status and sociodemographic characteristics of the patient population.

Recommendations

In the course of developing the tracer methodology, we encountered major limitations in available information that will affect planning and implementation of health services evaluation. Important issues relating to the use of the tracer methodology were identified also. Following are recommendations for both areas of concern.

INFORMATION NEEDS FOR HEALTH EVALUATION

A fundamental restructuring of national health information is needed. Technique and process orientation must give way to social utility and problem solving in data collection programs. Because data needs of all health-related activities cannot be met, however, priorities must be established.

National health and sociodemographic data must be restructured so that information from different agencies is compatible. In organizing the socioeconomic and clinical data for the first set of tracers, serious limitations were encountered in the availability, adequacy, and format of data collected by various federal agencies. Population information collected by such agencies as the Census Bureau, Labor Department, National Center for Health Statistics, and Office of Education, for example, should be capable of being easily reorganized so that the data are compatible and permit analysis of related characteristics.

Health data-collection programs should include information to

3

assess need, utilization, and cost for medical services. The National Center for Health Statistics conducts three periodic, operationally separate, nationwide surveys: the Health Records Survey, based on health records and utilization data obtained from hospitals and other institutions; the Health Interview Study, based on interviewing techniques to estimate prevalence of selected illnesses and disabilities, their functional impact, and, to a limited extent, the utilization and costs of particular health services; and the Health Examination Survey, in which clinical information for selected conditions is collected. Although each of the three sets of data is carefully organized and independently yields valuable information, their overall utility is lessened because they cannot be interrelated. Clinical data collected in the Health Examination Survey, for example, cannot be related to utilization data from the Health Records Survey or functional impact and cost data from the Health Interview Study. By including questions of utilization, cost, and functional impact in the Health Examination Survey, information useful for health planning and policy decisions could be collected.

Special efforts must be made to collect sociodemographic and medical data from critical, small-population subgroups. While it is important to have estimates of the prevalence of specific health problems in the general population, it is equally important to identify specific subgroups who are at high or low risk for certain disorders. Data are available, for example, to show that urban blacks in poverty have a high risk for contracting pulmonary tuberculosis. In considering the implications of these data for planning health services, it is essential to have similar data for other urban subpopulations, including poor whites and middle-income blacks and whites. The standard national sample will provide adequate data on three of these four groups, but because of the small size of the urban, middle-income, black population, a larger percentage of these individuals must be sampled to gather reliable data.

A minimal sociodemographic data base should be required of all health service programs. Physicians, program administrators, planners, and researchers need reliable sociodemographic data about the patient population served by their particular health services program. These are not research data. The same basic information required for evaluation is needed for delivering health services. The education of the head of a family, for example, is an indicator of the social position of the family that can be used by the physician delivering care, the administrator managing the practice, and the evaluator assessing various aspects of the delivery system. Most of the essential data need be collected only once—as people enroll in a program. At a minimum, these data should include complete name, home address, phone number, birthdate, sex, race, marital status, education of patient and head of family, occupation of patitent and head of family, health insurance carrier, welfare status, family composition, and source of previous medical care. These data, collected in the context of the delivery of health services, should be considered privileged, confidential communication between the patient and physician.

Structured record systems for collecting historical, physical, and laboratory data should be implemented in new delivery programs. Significant advances in the structuring of medical records have recently been made by development of the problem-oriented medical record. In its present form, or with modifications, this system of medical record-keeping allows for the collection and retrieval of problem-(tracer)-specific information. In delivery programs where options for innovation are present, it is now possible to utilize the problem-oriented record in gathering a data base for all patients. By combining the problem-oriented medical record and the tracer methodology for evaluation, a practical mechanism for ongoing medical evaluation can be tested.

FURTHER DEVELOPMENT OF THE TRACER METHODOLOGY

The tracer methodology should be tested in a variety of health service programs. To develop the tracer methodology further, it is necessary to test it in a sample of delivery systems. Pragmatic testing will provide experience necessary for revising the methodology and determining the extent to which the tracer method provides physicians and managers of health centers with information relevant to improving medical services.

The number and type of tracer sets should be expanded. Based on experience with one set of six tracers, we judge that the number of sets of tracers should be expanded to allow for better representation of age groups, types of disorders, and kinds of services. Additional tracers are needed to highlight special problems of youth and the elderly and to focus on the delivery of services to patients with emotional disorders. To develop additional tracer sets, criteria will have to be established and new data relating to epidemiology and the efficacy of care will have to be developed.

Summary

In their simplest definition, tracers are specific health problems that, when combined in sets, allow health care evaluators to pinpoint the strengths and weaknesses of a particular medical practice setting or an entire health service network by examining the interaction between providers, patients, and their environments.

The tracer concept was borrowed from the formal sciences. In physiology, for example, scientists use radioactive tracers to study how a body organ—such as the thyroid gland—handles a critical substance such as iodide. They measure how the thyroid takes up a minute amount of radioactive iodide and assume the organ handles natural iodide in the same manner.

In measuring the organ functions, or processes, of a health care body the tracers needed are discrete, identifiable health problems that flow through the system, each shedding light on how particular parts work, not in isolation, but in the system. The basic assumption remains the same; namely, how a physician or team of physicians routinely administers care for a common ailment or how a system identifies high-risk, pregnant women will be an indicator of the general quality of care and the efficacy of the system delivering that care.

In this study we have developed a set of six tracers, all common diseases treated by health care systems. Three of the tracers—iron-deficiency anemia; middle ear infection, including hearing loss; and visual disorders—were used to produce the evaluation found in Volume III of this study, *Contrasts in Health Status*. That evaluation focused on medical care given in five contrasting delivery systems. In

Volume I the outcomes of pregnancy, including infant death and birth weight, were used as tracers to evaluate the impact of medical care on infant mortality in certain groups within a large population.

CRITERIA FOR TRACERS

The value and reliability of evaluating health services by tracers rests on the selection of the tracers and the development of minimal care criteria against which the tracers can be compared.

Following are characteristics for selecting health problems to be used as tracers:

● *A tracer should have a significant functional impact on those affected.* Conditions that are unlikely to be treated or those that cause negligible functional impairment are poor choices.

● *Each should be relatively well defined and easy to diagnose in field and practice settings.* Dermatologic conditions, for example, require highly skilled professionals to diagnose and are difficult to screen on a mass basis. In contrast, it is relatively easy to delineate persons with iron-deficiency anemia.

● *Each should have a prevalency rate that is high enough to permit the collection of adequate data from a limited population sample.* If an adequate number of cases is not obtained, it is difficult to analyze important variables. For example, in comparing different organizations for providing care, evaluators must control for social and demographic characteristics of the patients.

● *The natural history of the condition should vary with utilization and effectiveness of medical care.* Ideally, in evaluating a delivery system, the tracer conditions should be sensitive to the quality and quantity of the service received by the patient.

● *The techniques of medical management of each condition should be well defined for at least one of the following processes: prevention, diagnosis, treatment, and rehabilitation or adjustment.* There is real danger in using outcome studies if it is unclear whether the provider can intervene in the natural course of the disease.

● *The effects of socioeconomic factors on each tracer condition should be understood.* Social, cultural, economic, and behavioral factors will introduce variations in the epidemiology of many morbidity conditions. The epidemiology should be relatively well understood. For instance, lead intoxication among children in urban areas is often caused by the ingestion of flaking, lead-based paint prevalent in slum housing. Thus, the medical delivery system that serves the ghetto and not the middle-income population is challenged to identify the population at risk and institute appropriate diagnostic, therapeutic, and preventive measures.

SELECTED TRACERS

In this study six tracers were selected by the above criteria. Together, the tracers form a set for evaluating health care received by a cross section of a typical service population. The tracers selected, and the segments of a population and health services they monitor, are:

● Middle Ear Infection and Associated Hearing Loss—The disease affects children of both sexes. Medical management requires screening, history taking, physical examination, hearing tests, drug prescription, education counseling, and follow-up. Treatment may also require that the child be referred to a hearing specialist.

● Vision Disorders—Visual disorders are common in persons of all ages. They are, however, especially useful for evaluating screening of persons between the ages of 5 and 25 years. Medical management requires screening and referral to specialists for corrective surgery, lenses, or both.

● Iron-Deficiency Anemia—Iron-deficiency anemia largely affects persons of both sexes who are under 5 years of age or over 25 years of age. Medical management requirements include prevention, screening, laboratory tests, drug treatment, health education counseling, and follow-up.

● Hypertension—Hypertension is found in persons of both sexes 25 years of age or older. Medical management consists of screening, history taking, physical examination, laboratory tests, drug treatment, and follow-up. In some instances, hospitalization is also required.

● Urinary Tract Infections—Urinary tract infections are most prevalent in females over 25 and males over 65. Medical management of urinary tract infections requires history taking, physical examination, drug treatment, and follow-up. In addition, some patients require hospitalization, specialty referral, or both.

● Cervical Cancer—Cervical cancer is a disease that strikes women in the 25-to-64-year-old range primarily. Medical management focuses mainly on screening and physical examinations. Other minimal medical processes are also highlighted by cervical cancer, however; these include history taking, laboratory tests, health counseling, referral to specialists, hospitalization, and follow-up.

When combined in sets, tracers provide a means of evaluating particular health services from two or more perspectives. For example, by combining iron-deficiency anemia and hearing loss—treatment for both includes screening and health education counseling—an evaluator can gain insight about a health center's performance in screening and counseling across the entire age and sex range of its patients.

EVALUATION AND CHANGE

The purpose of evaluation is twofold: to support good medical practice by identifying its efficacious and efficient elements, and to indicate areas of practice in need of improvement. In both instances the results of the evaluation must be geared to the needs of the persons responsible for managing the health services program.

By combining analyses of the set of six tracers developed in this study with census data and simple demographic information on the patients, basic strengths and deficiencies in specific aspects of a health care program can be identified, leading, where necessary, to changes in the organization and delivery of services. For example, in a hypothetical—although not farfetched—situation in which 25 percent of an enrolled high-risk population has not been screened for hypertension, only 11 percent of the estimated morbidity in the community has been identified, and significant differences exist between the care enrollees receive and the minimal care recommendations, the following steps seem appropriate:

1. Institute community case-finding efforts on a small population sample to determine the number of persons with high blood pressure not receiving care elsewhere in the community.
2. Restructure health-center procedures to obtain blood pressures on all high-risk enrollees.
3. Consider appropriate methods for administrative reorganization of follow-up procedures.

Reorganizing case-finding and screening procedures, the medical records system, and the management procedures for follow-up are only some of the things that quality assessment by tracers can do; it is a tool that will allow isolation of critical areas in the care process that indicate the kinds of services being delivered—their appropriateness, relative costs, and, most importantly, their impact on the well-being of the patient.

ONE

Development of the Tracer Method

THE STATE OF THE ART

Evaluation of health services is an emerging social, medical, and political issue. Increasing costs of medical services, growing government involvement in financing and delivering personal health services, heightened consumer sensitivity to the problems of quality care—all have contributed to its currency. As a result, more professional attention is now being devoted to quality assessment than ever before. Unfortunately, the methods available for evaluation are very primitive; they are neither reliable nor accurate. The reasons for this poor state of the art are complex. To a large extent they reflect the difficulties of assessing the quality of any complex social and personal service.

At the same time, the federal government and academic medical institutions have only recently begun to pay attention to issues in evaluating quality of care. For many years the nature of government research support and the structure of medical schools discouraged—in some cases, impeded—professional attention to the complex interaction of patients and medical practitioners.

In undertaking a comprehensive review of medical-care-assessment literature, Brook[1] screened 1,000 pertinent citations. He found that only 67 provided useful primary evaluation data. Furthermore, he noted that the authors of several studies that promise to advance our knowledge in these areas are just beginning to collect and analyze their data.

The idea of appraising the value of medical services and assessing their policy implications is not new. Sir William Petty, writing in England in the late seventeenth century, advocated state intervention on the basis of economic analyses to assure better medical services for the people, indicating that the Crown would profit from an investment aimed at lessening the effects of the plague.[2] In the mid-1800s, two pioneers in public health, Edwin Chadwick[3] and Lemuel Shattuck,[4] attempted to evaluate specific public program activities, to estimate their impact and cost, and to assess the implications of their findings for public policy. Using outcome data, Codman[5] began evaluating hospital services in the early 1900s. Although some specific issues have changed, the basic concerns remain pertinent to the problems that society faces today.

In their classic report *The Fundamentals of Good Medical Care,* issued almost 40 years ago, Lee and Jones[6] defined quality by eight "articles of faith": scientific basis for medical practice, prevention, consumer–provider cooperation, treatment of the whole individual, close and continuing patient–physician relationship, comprehensive and coordinated medical services, coordination between medical care and social services, and accessibility of care for all people. Today these remain unarguable goals for health services in the United States.

During the past decade and a half, the conceptual issues in evaluating health care programs have been restated many times.[7-18] The basic requirements for a pragmatic evaluation method include a statement of the objectives of the program, standards defining quality of care, data indicative of care delivered that can be compared to the standards, careful attention to the nature of the measurement units, assessment of the reliability of the analysis, consideration of the cost of the method, and a plan for integrating evaluation into the organization of health services.

Greater emphasis in evaluation has been placed on inpatient rather than outpatient, or ambulatory, medical services. Some techniques, however, have been applied in both settings. They include assessment of the skills and knowledge of physicians, judgments of the physician's method of practice by record review or direct observation, analyses of mortality and morbidity data as an indication of how care has affected the course of illnesses, analyses of medical service utilization factors, and assessment of patients' perceptions of, and satisfaction with, the care that has been received. No single method, however, is sufficient for a practical evaluation of the eclectic and complex organizations that provide personal health services.

Attempts to evaluate health care have been twice handicapped—
by the vexing question of what constitutes quality and by the technical problems inherent in specifying discrete and consistent measurement units. In evaluating hospital and ambulatory care, several investigators have focused on specific aspects of the medical care process to
develop measures indicative of overall quality.[19–25] These studies
employed medical audits that analyzed clinical records to assess the
management of particular conditions. In some, objective criteria were
formulated as standards for judging satisfactory performance.

The variability in disease severity, record quality, and organizational
structure encountered in outpatient settings make the evaluation of
ambulatory care particularly complex. Despite inherent difficulties,
however, several investigators used specific morbidity conditions as
a means of gathering data to analyze outpatient services. Selected
studies employing this approach in the evaluation of ambulatory
health services were reviewed; some examples are discussed below.

In a study of the medical clinic of a university hospital in the early
1960s, Huntley[26] analyzes charts for completeness of patient work-up
and proportion of abnormalities that were not followed up. More
than one fourth of the patients with a diastolic blood pressure of
100 mmHg or higher were given no special tests relevant to hypertension, and approximately one half of these patients had no diagnosis related to the cardiovascular system. Similar retrospective chart-
review techniques are applied to the emergency room setting by
Helfer[27] and Brook and Stevenson.[28] The latter study focuses on the
relation of process and outcome—measured by longevity, level of
symptoms, loss of work, hospitalization, and operations—for patients
with nonemergency gastrointestinal symptoms. The investigators conclude that only 27 percent of the 141 patients studied had received
effective care resulting in a positive outcome.

In a study of 296 patients with either urinary tract infection, hypertension, or an ulcerated lesion of the stomach or duodenum who were
treated at an emergency room, Brook[1] assesses five methods of evaluating health care. When the adequacy of the process of care is combined with judgments concerning outcome, Brook finds that the
quality of care appears to be acceptable for only 27 percent of the
cases.

Ciocco and colleagues[29] analyze services provided to 3,200 ambulatory patients who were seen for the first time by 16 different medical
groups. Utilizing case records as a source of data, they divide the diagnoses into 18 categories and evaluate the relations between complaint,

diagnosis, services and treatment, and the physicians' training and experience. Marked variations among the medical groups in the type and amount of service delivered are documented. After correcting for such patient characteristics as age, sex, and diagnosis, the investigators conclude that differences in the amount of training and specialty status of the physicians account for much of the variation.

In an attempt to evaluate the office practice of internists, Kroeger *et al.*[30] conducted a general review of office records for completeness and legibility. Abstracts of records in seven diagnostic categories were reviewed by ten physicians, who were asked to grade the quality of care rendered on a one-to-four scale. Despite the absence of guidelines or criteria and the lack of uniformity in backgrounds, general agreement is found among the physician-judges.

Morehead *et al.*[31,32] reviews charts to evaluate neighborhood health center performance in delivering preventive health care. Her analyses do not encompass clinical management or follow-up of potential pathology, but reflect the adequacy of the basic history, physical, and laboratory data and preventive care for adult medicine, obstetrics, and pediatrics. Using the performance of the medical-school-affiliated outpatient department as a standard, the study rates the neighborhood health centers above the hospitals in adult medicine and pediatrics and slightly below them in obstetrical care.

The studies that have been described utilized specific health problems or morbidity conditions as indicators of either process or outcome variables, or variables of process and outcome combined, in the delivery of ambulatory health services. The tracer methodology discussed in this chapter is a structured approach to the use of specific health problems in the appraisal of health services. The use of such indicators is not a new concept, but the manner in which the tracers were selected, the formulation of a set of tracers, the specification of criteria for care, and the concurrent assessment of provider and recipients represents a new approach to assessing personal health services. Underlying the tracer method is the basic assumption that how a physician or team of physicians routinely adminsters care for common ailments and what happens to the patients that receive that care will be an indicator of the general quality of the care delivered in that practice. Instead of focusing on the isolated patient or health professional, a set of tracers permits the consideration of a range of health service activities and the interactions between patient and health care provider. Further, the use of tracers allows for specificity in probing such questions as when, how, and by whom the condition was first identified; how and by whom it was or was not treated; and what the results of treatment were. Both patients and providers are essential to the evaluation; together they form the matrix through which the set of tracers is followed.

CRITERIA FOR EVALUATING CANDIDATE TRACERS

An important aspect of evaluation by tracers is the process by which those tracers are selected. The ultimate utility of the evaluation method is determined to a significant extent by the specific tracers selected for study. In an attempt to rationalize the decision-making process, we established the following criteria, presented in order of importance, for tracer selection. The decision process is shown in Figure 1. These criteria were used sequentially to select an initial set of six tracers from a larger list of morbidity and mortality conditions or preventive measures.

1. *A tracer should have a significant functional impact.* The over-riding purpose of the tracer approach is to focus on specific conditions that reflect the activities of health professionals. Conditions that are unlikely to be treated and those that cause negligible functional impairment are not useful.

2. *A tracer should be relatively well defined and easy to diagnose in both field and practice settings.* Dermatologic conditions have a clear functional impact. The difficulties, however, of defining clear-cut pathologic entities lessen their utility as tracers. In addition, screening for these conditions requires highly skilled professionals and is difficult to do en masse. In contrast, it is relatively easy to identify a population of patients with a hematocrit below a specified level. Using appropriate diagnostic tests, it is then possible to delineate further those with iron-deficiency anemia.

3. *Prevalence rates should be high enough to permit the collection of adequate data from a limited population sample.* If an adequate number of cases cannot be studied, it is difficult to evaluate even the most important variables in relation to the set of tracers. For example, in comparing different organizations for providing care, it is important to control for the social and demographic characteristics of their patients. This, in turn, requires a sufficiently large patient population.

4. *The natural history of the condition should vary with utilization and effectiveness of medical care.* Ideally, in evaluating a delivery sys-

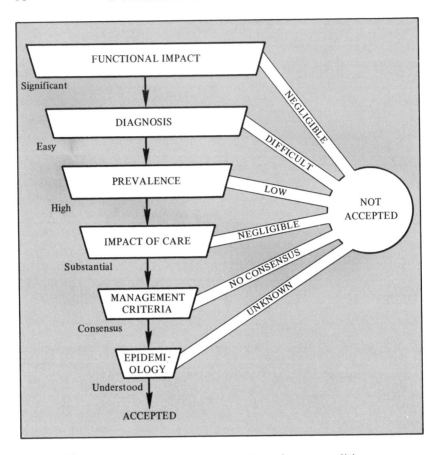

FIGURE 1   Decision tree for selection of tracer conditions.

tem, the conditions under study should be sensitive to the quality or quantity (or both) of the service received by the patient. It is inappropriate to use a genetic condition in which health services do not alter the progress of the disease.

5. *The techniques of medical management of the condition should be well defined for at least one of the following processes: prevention, diagnosis, treatment, or rehabilitation.* There is danger in using tracers as measures of the outcome of care if it is unclear whether the provider can intervene effectively in changing the course of the disease. There is now considerable controversy, for example, regarding the impact of oral hypoglycemic agents in adult onset diabetes mellitus. It is, therefore, of questionable value at this time to use diabetes as a tracer in

evaluating health services because it would be most difficult to agree upon minimal standards of care.

6. *The effects of nonmedical factors on the tracer should be understood.* Social, cultural, economic, and behavioral factors can influence the distribution of many morbidity conditions. Thus, the epidemiology of the tracer should be relatively well understood. For instance, lead intoxication among children in urban areas is often caused by the ingestion of flaking, lead-based paint prevalent in slum housing. For this reason the medical delivery system that serves the ghetto and not the middle-income population is challenged to identify the population at risk for lead intoxication and institute appropriate diagnostic, therapeutic, and preventive measures.

SELECTION OF A SET OF TRACERS

A set of six tracers—middle ear infection and hearing loss, visual disorders, iron-deficiency anemia, hypertension, urinary tract infections, and cervical cancer—was selected from a group of 15 candidate health problems according to the criteria presented in Figure 1. In all instances those conditions selected as tracers met the specifications outlined. As a set the six tracers can be used to evaluate the ambulatory care received by a cross section of the population. This set provides at least two individual tracers relevant to both sexes and the four age groups shown in Table1. In Table 2, a summary of the service functions highlighted* by these tracers is presented.

The activities of a health service delivery organization are categorized in five major groups. As shown in Table 2, each major activity is reflected by at least two different individual tracers. Thus, the varied activities of a delivery system are sampled by multiple tracers. In interpreting the analyses of an evaluation using the tracer method, similar evaluations for two or more tracers relative to a specific process strengthen the validity of the analyses. For example, if there is little or no screening for four or five tracers that highlight screening, we can assume with confidence that this medical process needs strengthening.

With the exception of middle ear infection, screening can easily be conducted for this set of tracers. Diagnostic criteria were felt to be

* The term "highlight" is used to indicate which service functions are best evaluated by each tracer and not whether a particular service function is relevant to the management of a given tracer.

TABLE 1   Age–Sex Groups Represented by Accepted Tracer Conditions

Age Group (years)	Tracer Conditions						
	Middle Ear Infection	Hear- ing Loss	Vision Defect	Iron- Deficiency Anemia	Hyper- tension	Urinary Tract Infection	Cervical Cancer
Female							
Under 5	+			+			
5–24	+	+	+				
25–64				+	+	+	+
65 or Over				+	+	+	
Male							
Under 5	+			+			
5–24	+	+	+				
25–64				+	+		
65 or Over				+	+	+	

relatively well defined for these conditions, although there remains some disagreement regarding specific criteria for hypertension, anemia, and significant bacteriuria. In addition, there is some vagueness associated with the etiology of serous otitis media. In general, prevalence rates were sufficiently high to expect an adequate number of cases, and there were substantial data to support the contention that medical care can intervene effectively in the natural history of these conditions.

A panel of consultants rejected nine potential tracers after applying the criteria shown in Figure 1. *Peptic disease* was eliminated because of the difficulty in screening for this condition, lack of strict diagnostic criteria, and the inability to judge the impact of a variety of different kinds of medical care on the natural history of the disease. Both *osteoarthritis* and *rheumatoid arthritis* were rejected because of the complexity of medical management and the difficulty of assessing the impact of treatment on the course of the illness. Logistical problems in screening for *cerebral vascular disease, coronary heart disease, rheumatic heart disease,* and *cancer of the rectum-colon* weighed heavily in rejecting these as tracers. Low prevalence rates for *cancer of the lung* and *cancer of the breast* were primary factors in rejecting those two conditions. There was consensus among the consultants that the variety of diagnostic entities encompassed under *chronic respiratory disease,* and the lack of impact of medical intervention limited the usefulness of this as a tracer condition.

TABLE 2   Aspects of the Process of Primary Ambulatory Health Care Highlighted by Accepted Tracer Conditions

Process Activities	Middle Ear Infection	Hearing Loss	Vision Defect	Iron-Deficiency Anemia	Hypertension	Urinary Tract Infection	Cervical Cancer
Prevention		+		+			
Screening		+	+	+	+		+
Evaluation							
History and physical exam	+				+	+	+
Laboratory				+	+	+	+
Other testing		+					
Management							
Chemotherapy	+			+	+	+	
Health counseling		+		+			+
Specialty referral	+	+	+			+	+
Hospitalization					+	+	+
Follow-up	+	+		+	+	+	+

APPLYING TRACER METHODOLOGY: AN EXAMPLE

The tracer method can be applied to a variety of organizations providing health services. It can be used to evaluate organizations, such as neighborhood health centers, that are responsible for providing care to a defined population; and it can be used to evaluate an individual physician who feels his responsibility is limited to those persons who come through his door.

In either case, the procedure does not vary greatly. It sets out to determine:

• How well the organization serves the people living in the community

• If appropriate screening and case-finding services are provided to the people who use the organization

• Whether the care that is provided meets minimal medical standards.

To illustrate the application of the tracer methodology, we have outlined a hypothetical community served by a hypothetical neighborhood health center. While some of the data we use in the illustration are real (developed in our pretests of the tracer method), some are not. These latter represent, rather, our generalized experience and "best guesses" in constructing a situation typical of those likely to be found by evaluators of urban health delivery systems.

A HYPOTHETICAL COMMUNITY

At the outset, two kinds of data are needed to define our hypothetical community and health center enrollees:

1. Current census figures, real or estimated, of demographic and socioeconomic characteristics of the population to be served by the neighborhood health center
2. Age and sex distributions of the persons enrolled in the neighborhood health center

Our community is located in the central city. Table 3 provides an overview of our community's sociodemographic characteristics. Its citizens are predominantly low-income blacks. The population density—number of persons living in the area—is high.

When we examine the age and sex distributions of our residents (Table 4), we find more than 40 percent of the population is under 25 years of age, almost 70 percent is under 45, and about 10 percent is over 65. These characteristics become crucial to our selection of tracers. We will want to use common ailments treated by the health system; we will want to examine routine, not unusual or exotic, care provided by the health center. Without knowing the predominant age and sex distributions of community residents, we cannot intelligently select tracer diseases that focus on routine care.

SERVING THE COMMUNITY

To find out how well our neightborhood health center serves our community, we need only compare the current Census data (Table 4) with a similar analysis of persons enrolled in and served by the health center. Our health center has 9,059 enrollees; enrollee distribution by age and sex is shown in Table 5.

In our sample analysis of how well the health center serves our community, we focus on two enrollee groups: males and females under

TABLE 3 Sociodemographic Characteristics of the Community Population[a]

Total population	42,390
Percent nonwhite	92%
Population density	37,849/mi²
Percent of persons below poverty level	22%
Percent of families below $5,000/year income	30%
Percent of adults less than 9 years education	29%

[a]Based on selected 1970 Census data.

15 years of age, and males 25 to 64. (In an actual evaluation, of course, we would examine all enrollee groups.)

From Table 6, we see that the health center serves about one fifth of all community residents. It is used to different extents, however, by the two age groups we have selected. Nearly one third of the children under 15 years of age are enrolled, but less than 15 percent of the 25-to-64-year-old males use the health center. To the administrator and governing board of the health center, this analysis provides a rather clear indication of total service provided to the community and, for planning, an indication of size of the community population whose needs have not been reached by the center. Most importantly perhaps, it points out a segment of the population—young to middle-age males—that has been underserved.

TABLE 4 Age–Sex Distribution[a] of the Community Population

Age Group (years)	Both Sexes		Males		Females	
	Number	%	Number	%	Number	%
Under 5	3,352	7.9	1,654	8.4	1,698	7.5
5–14	5,854	13.8	2,964	15.1	2,890	12.7
15–24	8,225	19.4	3,728	18.9	4,497	19.8
25–44	11,650	27.5	5,873	29.8	5,778	25.5
45–64	9,096	21.5	3,995	20.3	5,101	22.5
65 or over	4,213	9.9	1,466	7.4	2,747	12.1
TOTAL	42,390	100.0	19,680	99.9	22,711	100.1

[a]Based on selected 1970 Census data.

TABLE 5   Age–Sex Distribution of Community Neighborhood Health Center Enrollees

Age Group (years)	Both Sexes		Males		Females	
	Number	%	Number	%	Number	%
Under 5	1,295	14.3	640	16.9	655	12.4
5–14	1,657	18.3	852	22.5	805	15.3
15–24	1,954	21.6	750	19.8	1,204	22.9
25–44	2,673	29.5	998	26.3	1,675	31.8
45–64	1,085	12.0	401	10.6	684	13.0
65 or over	395	4.4	150	4.0	245	4.7
Total	9,059	100.1	3,791	100.1	5,268	100.1

SELECTING TRACERS

For the same two segments of the population—children under 15 and males 25 to 64—we will evaluate the health services provided by the center. To do this, we must select tracers and apply them to a sample of medical records. Which tracers we select are critical to the evaluation; ideally, they should consist of two sets (one for children and one for adults) of two or more tracers each. In that way we can view the services provided to each group from two or more perspectives and avoid the risk of isolating anomalous conditions. For simplicity in this illustration, however, we will use only one tracer for each group.

For the children, we chose middle ear infection, including associated hearing loss. As described in Chapter 2, minimal medical management for this ailment requires history taking, physical exami-

TABLE 6   Comparison of Community Population with Health Center Enrollees in Selected Age–Sex Groups

	Number of Persons		
	Community Population	Health Center Enrollees	% Community Population Enrolled
Total Population	42,390	9,059	21.4
Males, females 0–15 years	9,206	2,952	32.1
Males, 25–64 years	9,868	1,399	14.2

nation, medication, and follow-up. For the adult men, we chose hypertension—a disorder whose minimal medical management (see Chapter 5) includes screening.

We can estimate prevalence rates for both conditions in our community from a review of the literature. With reasonable assurance we know that at any given time about 15 percent of the children in our community will suffer from middle ear infection and about 23 percent of the men will suffer from hypertension. We can estimate therefore, that there will be approximately 1,380 children with middle ear infection and 2,270 males with hypertension in the community (see Table 7).

EFFECTIVENESS OF SCREENING

The results of our hypothetical review of the medical records of the adult males is summarized in Table 8. We collected the data according to the treatment criteria formulated for hypertension in Chapter 5 and found that 77 percent of the adult men had been screened for hypertension and that 258 cases had been identified, for a prevalence rate of 24 percent in the screened population.

From this analysis, we know:

● One fourth of the enrolled males were not screened.

● The same prevalence rate was found among screened patients as would be expected if they had been randomly selected from the enrollees, indicating that high-risk individuals had not been pinpointed for screening.

● The center is caring for only 11 percent of the estimated hypertensive adult males in the community.

TABLE 7   Estimated Prevalence of Middle Ear Infection and Hypertension in Selected Age–Sex Groups

Tracer	Community Population at Risk	Estimated Prevalence (%)	Estimated Number Cases in Community
Middle Ear Infection	9,206	15	1,380
Hypertension	9,868	23	2,270

TABLE 8   Detection of Hypertension in Health Center Enrollees

Cases	Estimated Cases in Community	Enrollees Screened at Health Center	Cases Detected at Health Center	Estimated Cases Detected in Community
Prevalence	2,270	1,077	258	258
Rate	23	77	24	11[a]

[a]Percent of total estimated adult males with hypertension in the community that were detected.

CONTENT OF CARE

When we reviewed the medical records of children with middle ear infection, we abstracted data based on the treatment criteria in Chapter 2. These criteria—like all treatment criteria in this volume— were formulated by practicing physicians and represent a consensus on *minimal* care.

On the basis of the abstracted data, we can evaluate the content of care received by the children. We can determine, for example:

1. How many children diagnosed as having middle ear infection had a minimal medical history taken and received the physical examination specified in the care standards.

2. How often appropriate drugs were prescribed.

3. In what proportion of cases was follow-up, including referral, carried out.

Table 9 displays hypothetical, but not atypical, data abstracted from medical records concerning the content of care provided to children with middle ear infection.

FEEDBACK AND IMPACT

In sum, the tracer method of evaluation requires the availability of community census data, simple demographic information on the population receiving care from a delivery system, and medical records. Analyses by age and sex of these data for the six-tracer set developed in this volume can locate specific deficiencies in a health care program. These should lead, in turn, to corrective changes in the organization and provision of services. In our hypothetical health center, for example, 25 percent of the enrolled high-risk population had not been

TABLE 9   Content of Care for Middle Ear Infection Compared to a Set
of Minimal Criteria

Process of Care	Percent Meeting Standards
Adequate medical history	50
Adequate physical examination	63
Appropriate medication	55
Appropriate follow-up/referral	70

screened for hypertension, and only 11 percent of the estimated morbidity in the community had been identified. Certain remedial actions
should be apparent to the administrator of the center:

• Institute community case-finding efforts on a small population
sample to determine the number of persons with high blood pressure
not receiving care elsewhere in the community.
• Restructure health center procedures to obtain blood pressures
on all high-risk enrollees.
• Consider use of structured medical records to obtain a minimal
data base for all patients.

On a more specific level, the center administrator will want to consider the information concerning appropriate drug therapy in middle
ear infection. Table 9 indicates that while 55 percent of the children
received appropriate medication, 45 percent did not. This is precisely
the kind of information that providers—solo physicians, health-center
administrators, medical directors, or consumer boards—need to improve care. First, it says that there may be something amiss in the way
a particular class of drugs—in this case, antibiotics—is prescribed, not
only for middle ear infection, but for other conditions as well. The
implication should then prod the responsible individual to ask: Is five
dollars' worth of prescription painkiller prescribed when 50 cents'
worth of aspirin would suffice? Are antibiotics routinely given for the
common cold? Are tranquilizers being used indiscriminately? and
other questions.

Improving case finding among high-risk groups, reorganizing medical
records and management procedures for follow-up, and pointing up
deficiencies in prescribing drugs are only some of the things that quality assessment by tracers can do. It is a tool allowing isolation and
analysis of critical areas in the care process that indicate the kinds of

services being delivered–their appropriateness, relative costs, and most importantly their impact on the well-being of the patient.

COSTS AND MANPOWER REQUIREMENTS

A few words about the costs and manpower requirements for evaluating by tracers are in order.

Costs, of course, will vary from practice to practice; they will be related, in large part, to the size of the health system to be evaluated, the clarity and condition of the medical records, the availability of competent personnel locally, prevailing wages in the area, and, ultimately, to the sharing of evaluation services, or teams, among many organizations of health providers. It seems doubtful that any single health delivery organization–except, perhaps, the very largest with multiple delivery points–can justify full-time evaluation staff.

Manpower requirements, however, offer a key to estimating the cost of evaluating a health center. Based on our experience in applying sets of tracers to evaluating live practice settings, we estimate the time required for a trained, four-member team (a leader and three chart abstractors) at a hypothetical health center as follows:

Planning and collecting community and enrollee data–team leader, one week, using protocol specifying needed data

Abstracting 1,000 medical records–three chart abstractors, four weeks, using precoded abstract forms

Processing data–one abstractor, two weeks, using established protocol for processing and editing

Analyzing and reporting data–team leader, four weeks, using protocol for analysis

The estimate is based on several assumptions. First, the team leader, or director, is knowledgeable of evaluation and basic statistical theory as well as aware of medical processes and organizational options for service delivery. Second, the other team members have had working experience (perhaps as nurses or paramedics) in health delivery, are conversant with health care jargon, and familiar with normal routines in providing health services. Third, the precoded abstract forms and protocols for abstracting and analysis have been previously developed. And, finally, the health delivery unit will provide assistance in identifying and pulling records to be examined.

REFERENCES

1. Brook RH: A study of methodologic problems associated with assessment of quality of care. Department of Medical Care and Hospitals, Johns Hopkins University (PhD dissertation) 1972
2. Petty Sir William: Of Lesening ye Plagues of London (1667), The Economic Writings of Sir William Petty. Edited by CH Hull. Cambridge, The University Press, 1899, p 109
3. Chadwick E: Report on the Sanitary Conditions of the Labouring Population of Great Britain, 1842. Edinburgh, Edinburgh University Press, 1965 p 443.
4. Shattuck L: Report of the Sanitary Commission of Massachusetts, 1850. Forward by Charles Edward Amory Winslow. Cambridge, Harvard University Press, 1948 p 321
5. Codman EA: A study in hospital efficiency: The first five years. Boston, Thomas Todd Co, 1916
6. Lee RI, Jones LW: The Fundamentals of Good Medical Care. Chicago, University of Chicago Press, 1933 (Publication of the Committee on the Costs of Medical Care, No 22)
7. Donabedian A: A guide to medical care administration, Vol. II: Medical Care Appraisal–Quality and Utilization. New York, The American Public Health Association, Inc, 1969
8. Hopkins CE (ed): Outcomes Conference I–II: Methodology of identifying, measuring and evaluating outcomes of health service programs, systems and subsystems. Rockville, Md, Department of Health, Education, and Welfare, Public Health Service, Health Services and Mental Health Administration, 1969
9. Altman I, Anderson AJ, Barker K: Methodology in Evaluating the Quality of Medical Care. Pittsburgh, University of Pittsburgh Press, 1969
10. Klein BW: Evaluating outcomes of health services: An annotated bibliography Los Angeles, School of Public Health, California Center for Health Services Research, University of California, 1970 (working paper No 1)
11. Donabedian A: Evaluating the quality of medical care. Milbank Mem Fund Q 44(3):166–206, 1966
12. Donabedian A: Promoting quality through evaluating the process of patient care. Med Care 6(3):181–202, 1968
13. Shapiro S: End result measurements of quality of medical care. Milbank Mem Fund Q 45(Part I):7–30, 1967
14. United States Department of Health, Education, and Welfare. Vital and Health Statistics: Conceptual Problems in Developing an Index of Health. Rockville, Md. 1966 (PHS Publication No. 1000, Series 2, No. 17)
15. Kelman HR, et al: Strategy and tactics of evaluating a large-scale medical care program. Med Care 7:79–85, 1969
16. Kerr M, et al: Defining, measuring and assessing the quality of health services. Public Health Rep 84:415–424, 1969
17. Kelin MW, et al: Problems of measuring patient care in the out-patient department. J Health Human Behav 2:138–153, 1961
18. Donabedian A: The evaluation of medical care programs. Bull NY Acad Med 44(2):117–124, 1968

19. Lembcke PA: Medical auditing by scientific methods. JAMA 162:646–655, 1956

20. Eislee CW, Slee VN, Hoffman RG: Can the practice of internal medicine be evaluated? Ann Intern Med 44:144–161, 1956

21. Payne BC: Continued evaluation of a system of medical care appraisal. JAMA 201:126–130, 1967

22. Falk IS, Schonfeld HK, Harris BR, et al: The development of standards for audit and planning of medical care. I. Concepts, research design, and the content of primary physician's care. Am J Public Health 57:1118–1136, 1967

23. Schonfeld HK, Falk IS, Lavietes PH, et al: The development of standards for the audit and planning of medical care: Pathways among primary physicians and specialists for diagnosis and treatment. Med Care 6:101–114, 1968

24. Schonfeld KH, Falk IS, Lavietes PH, et al: The development of standards for the audit and planning of medical care: Good pediatric care—Program content and method of estimating needed personnel. Am J Public Health 58: 2097–2110, 1968

25. Schonfeld HK, Falk IS, Sleeper HR, et al: The content of good dental care: Methodology in formulation for clinical standards and audits, and preliminary findings. Am J Public Health 57:1137–1146, 1967

26. Huntley RR: The quality of medical care: Techniques and investigation in the outpatient clinic. J Chronic Dis 14(6):630–642, 1969

27. Helfer RE: Estimating the quality of patient care in a pediatric emergency room. J Med Educ 42:244–248, 1967

28. Brook RH, Stevenson RL: Effectiveness of patient care in an emergency room. New Eng J Med 283:904–907, 1970

29. Ciocco A, Hunt H, Altman I: Statistics on clinical services to new patients in medical groups. Public Health Rep 65:99–115, 1950

30. Kroeger HH, Altman I, Clark DA, et al: The office practice of internists. I. The feasibility of evaluating quality of care. JAMA 193:121–126, 1965

31. Morehead, MA: Evaluating quality of medical care in the neighborhood health center program of the office of economic opportunity. Med Care 8:118–131, 1970

32. Morehead MA, Donaldson RS, Seravalli MR: Comparisons between OEO neighborhood health centers and other health care providers of ratings of the quality of health care. Am J Public Health 61:1294–1306, 1971

Middle Ear Infection and Associated Hearing Loss

SUMMARY

The combined tracer of middle ear infection and conductive hearing loss highlights an array of health services in the pediatric age group. Screening and case finding for hearing loss is indicated in the general pediatric population and especially in children with recurrent middle ear infection. The diagnosis, treatment, and follow-up of middle ear infection exemplifies, in general, how acute infectious conditions are managed in this population. The appropriateness and completeness of the history and physical examination and the use of antibiotics and symptomatic chemotherapy can be explored. There is sufficient need for specialty referral to be able to assess how referrals are managed and integrated into the primary care system.

CLASSIFICATION

Middle ear infections can be classified on the basis of etiology and pathogenesis into four categories: acute serous otitis media, acute purulent otitis media, chronic serous otitis media, and chronic suppurative otitis media. The classification "serous" includes a spectrum of middle ear infections characterized by serous, as well as mucous (often referred to as exudative otitis media or "glue ear" in the chronic stage), nonpurulent fluid in the middle ear.

29

EPIDEMIOLOGY

Age and Sex General-practice surveys describe a significant range among urban children at highest risk of infection; where some data report peak annual incidence rates in children aged 3–4 and 6–7, 60 percent of one urban study population experienced their index attack before age 2. In contrast, a study of ear disease and hearing sensitivity by Eagles *et al.* on elementary school children in Pittsburgh reports a lower proportion of children with abnormal findings in the youngest age group, with an increase at age 5, maintained to 10, and followed by a steady decline. Differential rates of infection by sex are shown to be of negligible statistical significance.

Race The significance of this variable would appear to be discounted by the striking intraracial differential in prevalence rates recorded in the literature. The incidence of middle ear pathology in Caucasians living in Wasilla, Alaska, is three times as high as among Alaska teachers' children, and dramatic variations have been found in incidence levels between neighboring Eskimo villages and neighboring Indian tribes. Studies have shown poor Appalachian Caucasians and Eskimos to be comparable high-risk groups, with rough prevalence estimates of acute otitis media of 20 percent and 33 percent, respectively, in the pediatric age group.

Seasonal Variation Incidence of middle ear infection in the period December/January through March/April is often reported to be twice to three times as high as rates recorded in July/August. This pattern is consistently reported from studies of differing population groups in contrasting climates and is positively correlated with the incidence of upper respiratory infection.

Socioeconomic Status Although definitive research is lacking, the literature indicates that in selected populations rates of middle ear disease and socioeconomic status may be inversely related. Based on a crude rating of socioeconomic status within an Indian tribe, the class designated "poor" experienced a rate of aural disease six times as high as was found in the class rated "good." Investigators studying the middle ear disease problem among Indians and Eskimos consistently isolate poverty-related conditions—poor hygiene, sanitation, housing, and diet—as predisposing factors explaining the high prevalence of middle ear pathology in these populations.

FUNCTIONAL IMPACT

Hearing Loss The most reliable information available on the extent of hearing impairment caused by middle ear disease comes from a recent study conducted on a population who had suffered acute otitis media 5–10 years previously. Seventeen percent of that group suffered a hearing loss of 20 decibels (db) or more in at least two frequencies.

Educational Handicap Recent studies suggest that as little as a 15-db hearing loss can lead to backwardness in such basic subjects as arithmetic and English. Children with impaired hearing have also been found more likely to be delayed admission to school and twice as likely to repeat a grade as children with normal hearing. In a study of children suffering from fluctuating hearing loss accompanying chronic otitis media, educational handicaps are found: These children are deficient in vocabulary acquisition, articulation skills, ability to receive and express ideas through spoken language, use of grammar and syntax, and auditory memory skills.

A MINIMAL-CARE PLAN FOR MIDDLE EAR INFECTIONS IN CHILDREN

I. Evaluation

 A. *History.* (1) Presenting symptoms and duration; (2) occurrence of: pain in ears, draining ears, fever, hearing problems; (3) prior treatment for this episode; (4) specify allergies, history of previous middle ear infection, operations on ear, nose, or throat if not a part of a past history previously recorded.
 B. *Physical examination.* Description of (1) temperature; (2) abnormal auditory canals; (3) abnormal tympanic membranes; (4) abnormal cervical lymph nodes; (5) abnormal pharynx.

II. Diagnosis

Differentiate between suppurative and nonsuppurative (serous) otitis media, and between acute and chronic suppurative otitis media.

III. Management

All drugs are prescribed in acceptable dosages adjusted to the individual patient, contraindications are observed, and patients are monitored for common side effects according to information detailed in *AMA Drug Evaluations, 1971*. Fixed-dosage combinations should not be used for initial therapy.

    A. *Treatment of suppurative otitis media.* (1) Antimicrobial drugs: The duration of treatment should be 7–10 days. In general, multiple antimicrobials should not be used. Under 6 years of age, ampicillin is drug of choice. If patient is allergic to penicillin, use erythromycin. Six years or older, use penicillin G, one of its derivatives, or tetracycline. Tetracycline should not be used when the patient is pregnant. If patient is allergic to penicillin, use erythromycin. (2) Nasal decongestant: ephedrine class of compounds by oral route; no combinations.

    B. *Treatment of nonsuppurative (serous) otitis media.* (1) Use antimicrobials as described above if there is evidence of concomitant suppurative infection; (2) use antihistamines only if there is evidence of allergy; (3) nasal decongestant: ephedrine class of compounds by oral route; no combinations.

    C. *Follow-up.* (1) Re-examine 10–14 days after treatment initiated; (2) evaluate hearing if there are repeated infections or evidence of hearing loss.

    D. *Referral.* (1) To otolaryngologist if there is persistent infection or effusion not responsive to three courses of treatment; (2) to otolaryngologist for recurrent infection and decision for tonsilectomy and adenoidectomy.

CLINICAL ASPECTS

Salient features of the clinical aspects of middle ear infection are summarized in the material below.[1-5] There is some disagreement as to the diagnostic categories of middle ear infections. As used here, otitis media will be classified by the following characteristics: (a) acute and chronic suppurative otitis media, and (b) acute and chronic nonsuppurative otitis media.

    Acute and chronic infections of the upper respiratory tract are the most common etiologic factors in the development of acute and

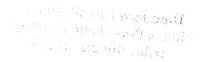

chronic suppurative middle ear infections. Recent microbiological and serological surveys of middle ear infection report that the antecedent upper respiratory infections are usually viral in origin. In the pediatric age group the most important viral agents are the respiratory syncytial virus in infants up to 2 years old, parainfluenza virus types 1, 2, and 3 in ages 3 through 6, and sporadic epidemics of rhinovirus. Although it is felt by many authorities that viral infections are the prime causative agents, bacterial infection is soon superimposed and accounts for the majority of the common acute and chronic suppurative infections. There is some disagreement concerning the bacterial agents that most commonly complicate middle ear disease; *Pneumococcus,* beta-hemolytic *Streptococci, Hemophilus influenzae,* and *Staphylococcus aureus* are most frequently implicated.

The primary pathologic process is a blockage of the eustachian tube resulting from an inflammatory process. The resultant negative pressure in the middle ear causes secretions (initially sterile) to accumulate. At this early stage of acute middle ear disease otologic examination reveals a dull tympanic membrane showing possible signs of mild inflammation. Characteristic symptoms, which increase in intensity with duration of illness, include intermittent or continuous earache, a feeling of fullness in the ear, fever and malaise, and sporadic hearing loss. With the invasion of virulent bacteria into the middle ear, acute suppuration soon occurs, and the eardrum appears markedly abnormal in color and position. At this stage both severe throbbing pain and marked hearing loss are experienced. If pressure increases from pus accumulation, the eardrum may rupture, discharging a mixture of blood and pus and relieving pain. If the infection is controlled at this stage, the inflammatory swelling of the eustachian tube normally subsides and symptoms disappear. In severe cases with recurrent attacks and inadequate care, a potentially destructive stage of disease, chronic suppurative otitis media, may develop. In that case the eardrum is permanently perforated and dangerous complications may result. Recurrent purulent discharge and residual hearing impairment of increasing severity are cardinal symptoms of this chronic stage.

In addition to impaired hearing, which varies greatly in intensity with the severity of reaction, other typical clinical signs of chronic middle ear disease include (a) an abnormal eardrum, usually retracted and rarely bulging, that is frequently scarred, thickened, and opaque or increasingly transparent in early stages, ranging in color from a faint yellowish to a dark blue; (b) fluid in the middle ear, ranging from amber watery serum to gray gelatinous masses of high viscosity; and

(c) chalky white appearance of the malleus and prominence of the short process. The patient may complain of a full feeling in the ear and mild earache or suffer low-pitched tinnitus and vertigo. Rarely does decreased hearing sensitivity, which also may go unnoticed in mild cases, present itself as the only symptom. When serous otitis media is a result of acute causative factors (commonly, viral or bacterial infections of the upper respiratory tract), it is usually of comparatively short duration. When the infection subsides, the serum collection should absorb or drain out through the eustachian tube, and the appearance of the eardrum and hearing should return to normal. The secretory conditions of a more complex etiology are more difficult to treat successfully. Protracted cases are commonly caused by conditions such as allergy and endocrine disorders or chronic nasopharyngeal disease that affect water balance in body tissues. In cases where treatment is not directed to these underlying causes, the condition may become chronic and produce fibrous adhesions in the middle ear and other irreversible destructive processes that can directly lead to permanent impairment of hearing.

EPIDEMIOLOGY*

AGE

The prevalence and incidence of middle ear infections by age is relatively well documented. Although some discrepancy appears in reports on the age group at highest risk, a general epidemiologic pattern is consistently reported in the literature: Onset of middle ear disease (both acute and serous†) commonly occurs in early childhood, with highest morbidity rates found among children under 10 years.

Several urban studies based on hospital clinical records appear to isolate the preschool population as the high-risk age group for experiencing acute middle ear infections. In an early study by Nielson in

---

* Presented, in part, at the National Otitis Media Conference, Dallas, Texas, May 15–17. 1970. McEldowney D, Kessner DM: The epidemiology of otitis media, Otitis Media: Proceedings of the National Conference. Edited by A Glorig, KS Gerwin. Springfield, Illinois, Charles C Thomas, 1972

† As used below, "acute" middle ear disease or otitis media denotes suppurative (involving pus formation) disease; "serous" denotes a nonsuppurative process. When no diagnostic information is available the condition will be referred to simply as "otitis media" or "middle ear infection."

Copenhagen[6] of cases of acute otitis media seen in city hospitals, over half of the patients are 4 years old and under; the youngest children are particularly susceptible to middle ear infection. Similarly, clinical records from the Johns Hopkins Comprehensive Child Care Program* reveal that among 1,700 annual cases of otitis media, as many as 80 percent per quarter occur in children 4 years and under. Feingold *et al.*[7] studied children with acute middle ear infection seen at Boston City Hospital and report that 62 percent of the cases occur in children 2 years and under.

General practice surveys appear to define a wider range of high-risk ages. Fernandez and McGovern[8] conclude from their investigation of a series of cases with serous otitis media treated in general practice that 68 percent of the children are first seen for treatment between the ages of 5 and 8, a high-risk age range for serous otitis media that Yunginger's[9] independent research confirms. Yet Fernandez determines that in 74 percent of cases the disease process is established before age 4. Lemon's[10] study on serous otitis media in Philadelphia produces contrasting results: He determines that 70 percent of his series experienced onset of symptoms between 4 and 7 years, with a sharp peak rate at 6. This age pattern is strikingly similar to incidence data from the Medical Research Council's[11] study on acute otitis media in general practices in Great Britain. This study documents annual incidence for 2-year-olds of 14 percent, climbing to a peak of 20 percent at 6, and sharply declining among older children.

The Medical Research Council's data set incidence levels of 12 percent for children 10 years and under. Two subsequent British studies[12, 13] on acute otitis media in general practice produce comparable annual incidence figures on this age group of 10 percent and 15 percent, respectively, while documenting a significantly different incidence pattern within this age group. In a 10-year general practice survey, Fry[12] finds the highest annual incidence rates of acute otitis media among 4-year-olds, with children 4–8 experiencing a high risk of infection. In a Liverpool general practice studied by Lowe *et al.*,[13] an age distribution with two incidence peaks is observed, the first occurring in the second 6 months of life and the second in the 5- to 6-year age group. In his study of South Carolina children with acute otitis media, Brownlee *et al.*[14] documents a comparable pattern in the relative frequency of attacks by age.

Official morbidity statistics from general practice in Great Britain[15]

* R. H. Drachman, personal communication, November 1969.

provide a further source on age patterns: When children are grouped as 0–1, 1–5, and 5–14 years, the youngest group has an approximately 50 percent higher annual patient consulting rate than the middle group and approximately 30 percent higher than the oldest children. Reed and Brody's[16] study of middle ear disease in a Caucasian working-class practice in Anchorage, Alaska, reveals high incidence among children under 10; but of the children whose index attack could be dated, the initial episode occurred in 42 percent before their first birthday and in 60 percent before their second. It is noteworthy that in several independent studies of patients with both serous and acute middle ear infections seen in general practice, well over 50 percent of the total cases are found in children 10 years and under.[8,9,17,18]

While general practice surveys reach a concensus that the large majority of cases of otitis media occur in children under 10, divergence of opinion exists on whether high-risk ages are the preschool or early school years. At least one urban study[19] fails to find relationships between morbidity and age in children 2 through 16 with otitis media. School surveys, because of the limited age range involved, do not offer a solution to this problem; nevertheless, two are worthy of mention. A hearing survey conducted in Vancouver[20] on an elementary school population records the highest incidence rates of serous otitis media in children enrolled in grades one through three, a rate of disease averaging two to three times as high as is found in grade five. A comprehensive study of ear disease and hearing sensitivity was conducted by Eagles et al.[21] on elementary school children in Pittsburgh. An analysis of the age at which signs of middle ear pathology were first reported shows an apparently lower proportion of children with abnormal findings in the youngest age group, with an increase at age 5, maintained to 10, and followed by a steady decline. But it is significant that 42 percent of the total cases found in children participating longest in the survey (i.e., on the average the youngest upon entry) were discovered at their initial exam. Eagles concludes that preschool as well as very early school years are likely to be high-risk ages for the onset of middle ear disease. However, when prevalence of middle ear disease from this study[22] is analyzed by age (cohorts 5 and 6), no trend is apparent.

Studies of acute otitis media conducted among Alaska native populations more consistently describe a very early age of onset of pathology and highest incidence of infections in the preschool age group. Brody[23] concludes that middle ear disease appears established in approximately one third of the Eskimo village population by age 2. D. D. Beal* estimates an even higher morbidity rate among the very young: Approximately 60 percent of all Alaska native children have at least one episode of acute middle ear infection in the first year of life. In a study in the Bethel area,[24] it is determined that the median age of the first episode is 6 months. A cohort study[25] of Eskimo children, followed from birth to 4 years, reveals that 89 percent of the cases of acute otitis media during the 4 study years occur in children under 2. In contrast, a recent study of Eskimos on Baffin Island[26] reports that there is no significant decrease in the prevalence of active ear disease with age when children 0–4 years old are compared with those 5–9. Similarly, Reed and Dunn[27] find that after the first year of life, little change in age incidence is apparent.

A parallel pattern of onset and recurrence has been documented among the American Indians. In a study of Texas Indians,[28] it is reported that children diagnosed with acute otitis media usually suffered ear drainage in the first year of life. Early age of onset is also noted among reservation Indians in British Columbia;[29] in 64 percent of the cases of acute otitis media where the index case could be dated, patients suffered their first acute infection before age 5. These results are confirmed by Zonis'[30] observations among Indians in the Southwest. There is, however, one group of investigators[31] that challenges the findings of any clear age pattern in rates of middle ear disease among American Indians. Also, in a report on the clinical impression of medical personnel working with the Indians, Jaffee[32] states that the common age for the index episode of acute otitis media is 3–6 months.

Some investigators[11, 33] attempt to account for the age distribution of serous and acute middle ear infections on the basis of physiologic differences, which act as predisposing factors to tubal obstruction, in the upper respiratory tract of young children and in the greater risk in early childhood of cross infection. It appears that severity, duration, and/or frequency of episodes of acute middle ear infection, and *not* age of onset, is positively correlated with risk of subsequent hearing impairment.[24, 25,27,29,33, 34] Yet a pattern of increased susceptibility to reinfection with each new episode often has been documented,[27,35] and at least one investigator[12] believes recurrences more likely the earlier the index attack.

---

* Personal communication, December 1969.

SEX

It is known that males generally have higher infection rates than females in the pediatric age group. A review of the literature for incidence and prevalence rates of middle ear pathology by sex uncovers several reports documenting a slightly higher risk among males.

One investigator in Sweden[36] finds a disproportionate number of males under 3 years experiencing acute middle ear infections with no apparent sex trend in older children. Among cases of acute otitis media seen in Copenhagen hospitals,[6] 56 percent are males; and this slight differential risk is consistent in all age groups. In Feingold's[7] investigation of cases with acute middle ear disease seen at Boston City Hospital, male cases constitute 61 percent of his population. An Alaska-based urban study[16] documents a slightly higher risk of infection among Caucasian males. A recent study of acute middle ear disease among native preschool children of Guam[37] reports that males experience significantly higher rates than females for such symptoms as draining ear and earache; the majority of conductive hearing losses among school children (attributable to middle ear disease) are also found among males.

Only Yunginger's study[9] of a series of children with serous otitis media reports dramatic differences by sex: Middle ear effusion is observed in twice as many males as females. In stark contrast, the Vancouver study[15] of a larger and more representative sample of the elementary school population documents no significant variation by sex in rates of serous otitis media. This conclusion is also reached in two British studies,[11,13] documenting the epidemiologic patterns of acute otitis media.

Reed's studies of middle ear pathology among Eskimo children have revealed no clear sex pattern. He reports a slightly higher percentage of males experiencing draining ears in one study,[25] whereas no sex-related differences in rates of pathology can be demonstrated after the first year of life in a later investigation[27] One study on South Dakota Indians[31] reveals no sex differential in rates of acute otitis media.

The literature thus provides no concensus on the importance of sex as an epidemiologic parameter. Using available information, the tentative conclusion must be drawn that sex is unlikely to be a major determinant of morbidity rates.

RACE

Few studies have explored the relationship of race to the prevalence, incidence, and severity of middle ear disease. Although the existing studies of this condition cover a wide range of population groups, few attempt interracial comparisons. Much of the past research has focused on American Indians and Alaska natives, while urban Negroes have apparently not been studied in this connection. Moreover, it is difficult to compare the various studies on contrasting racial groups because of differences in sampling procedures, screening criteria, and lack of control for such variables as socioeconomic status.

Because of the disproportionately high rates of middle ear disease among American Indians and Eskimos, it has been suggested that genetic differences in skull and middle ear shape and/or the production of cerumen might be causative factors.* One study[38] shows that there are genetically determined differences in cerumen type, but no studies that definitely relate these biologic phenomena to differences in rates of middle ear pathology were found. The usefulness of studies of middle ear anatomy in high-risk populations has been emphasized.[30,37,39] Johnson[40] reports that clinical experience among the Indians has failed to reveal any anatomical explanation for the high morbidity rate in this population. Contrasting findings come from a study of cleft uvulae among American Indians reported by Jaffee.[32] This anomaly is shown to occur significantly more frequently in Indians, and among Indian children with major cleft uvulae the rates of otitis media are twice as high as in the normal Indian population. The need for further evaluation in this area is also illustrated by a more recent report by Jaffee *et al.,*[41] who examine the tympanic membranes of newborn Indians within the first 2 days of life. Eighteen percent have either completely or partially immobile drums on examination. Follow-up studies lead to the conclusion that two out of three neonates with poor drum mobility develop otitis media before their first birthday. Delayed ventilation of the middle ear spaces after birth has also been observed to occur often among Eskimo infants.† Although such findings suggest that an anatomical factor such as middle ear shape might be involved, Jaffee finds that two of the three factors positively correlated with immobile drums are prematurity and maternal complications during pregnancy. Another biologic as-

*J. Brody, personal communication, May 1969.
† R. Pumphrey, personal communication, May 1969.

pect yet to be extensively treated in the literature is the relevance of immunologic deficiencies as determinants of high risk. Dolowitz[28] fails to find a relationship between otitis media and deficient immunologic mechanisms.

In 1967 otitis media was documented as the leading reportable disease among American Indians,[42] with a prevalence rate for all ages of 8,099 per 100,000. Individual investigators studying middle ear disease among American Indians confirm these striking statistics. In an otoscopic survey of Navajo school children, Johnson[40] observes a prevalence of chronic otitis media of over 7 percent; an additional 8 percent of the population exhibit signs of past pathology. Among Indian school children in South Dakota,[31] a combined prevalence rate for acute and chronic otitis media of 30 percent is reported. Zonis[30] conducted a complete prevalence survey of middle ear disease in a White Mountain Apache community and observes a similarly severe morbidity experience: Of the total population, 8.3 percent has chronic otitis media, with an additional 13 percent showing signs of past infection. A comparable general prevalence survey conducted among Indians on the Mt. Currie Reservation, British Columbia,[29] reports that 13.7 percent of the population has middle ear disease. A total of 45 percent are known to have had at least one episode of severe infection in their lives, and over 31 percent are recorded as having an abnormal audiogram (15 db or more loss in the speech range, American Standard for Audiometers (ASA), 1951). Significantly, Zonis[30] and Dolowitz[28] independently observe that some neighboring tribes experience a far lower rate of middle ear disease, i.e., that apparently a marked *intra*-racial variation in morbidity experience exists.

Otitis media constitutes a health problem of similar if not of greater proportions among Alaska natives. According to Public Health Service data,[42] prevalence rates for 1967 were 5,879 per 100,000 for all ages, with independent studies conducted among native populations recording even higher rates. Beal reports that 10 percent of the total Eskimo population suffers from chronic otitis media with a significant hearing loss in one ear, and that approximately 60 percent of the Eskimo children experience at least one acute infection during the first year of life. Another study[25] reveals that 64 percent of Eskimo children have at least one episode of otorrhea during 4 years of observation, with 31 percent recording a hearing deficit of 26 db or more (any frequency 500–4,000 Hz, International Organization for Standardization (ISO), 1964). A more recent investigation[27] documents a 1-year prevalence of 43 percent among Eskimo children under age 10: Of the children able to undergo audiometric testing, 27 percent record hearing losses of 26 db or more. While these figures are indeed dramatic, the fact that medical personnel[43,44] have noted a wide variation in prevalence and severity of middle ear disease between neighboring villages indicates that significant intraracial differences in morbidity experience also occur within Eskimo populations.

Three Alaska-based studies provide interracial comparative data. The first records a striking interracial differential in prevalence of pathology for all ages.[44] The pertinent results are given in Tables 1 and 2.

In a more recent study, Eskimos are compared with Euro-Canadians.[26] Among Eskimo children 31 percent show evidence of active acute middle ear disease and hearing loss, while none of the Caucasian children screened show evidence of either ear disease or hearing loss. The inadequate size of the Caucasian sample precludes firm conclusions, however.

A most useful study incorporating both inter- and intraracial comparisons was conducted by Brody *et al.*[43] in which various Alaskan and non-Alaskan population segments are compared by racial stock for the prevalence of draining ears and hearing loss. Tables 3 and 4 record these results.

What is striking in these findings is that although the Eskimos experienced a higher rate of draining ears and severe hearing impairment, the Caucasians sampled from Wasilla also experience a very high percentage of cases of otorrhea; the rate is three times as high as in the other Caucasian groups sampled. One observation made by Brody is especially relevant to this discussion: While approximately one third of the Eskimo population studied suffers from severe infection and frequent attacks of middle ear disease, the remaining two thirds seem

TABLE 1 Percent of Alaskans with Abnormal Tympanic Membrane[a]

Race	Percent
Eskimo	57.9
Indian	43.5
Native, mixed	49.2
Caucasian	36.4
ALL	53.3

[a]Defined as presence of perforation, scarring, retraction, or inflammation.
Source: Hayman and Kester.[44] Reprinted by permission.

TABLE 2   Percent of Alaskans with Abnormal Hearing[a]

Race	Percent
Eskimo	33.7
Indian	23.3
Native, mixed	20.8
Caucasian	14.3
ALL	27.8

[a]20-db or more loss in two frequencies, ASA 1951.
Source: Hayman and Kester.[44] Reprinted by permission.

to remain unaffected, comprising an intraracial group with a contrasting low risk of infection.

In discussing this morbidity condition, Deuschle[3] draws a parallel between the prevalence and severity of otitis media among American Indians and Alaska natives with the high rates found among poor Appalachian Caucasians in Kentucky. Based on data from a Martin County, Kentucky, study,[45] which records rough prevalence estimates in the infant population (0–2 years) of 20 percent for acute infections, 5 percent for chronic, and prevalence of all ear disorders of 336.4 per 1,000, the populations appear of comparably high risk although of contrasting racial stock.

Possible relevant factors (e.g., socioeconomic status) in the relationship of race to the prevalence, incidence, and severity of otitis media are often ignored. No material regarding the relationship of race to rates of serous otitis media is available, and at the present time only tentative conclusions may be inferred from the available information on acute otitis media. Because of the significant differential rates reported within racial groups and comparable rates documented between groups, race appears not to be an important factor influencing morbidity rates for acute middle ear disease.

SOCIOECONOMIC FACTORS

Definitive studies on the relationship of socioeconomic factors to the prevalence and severity of suppurative middle ear disease are currently lacking; in fact, only one study relating serous otitis media to these factors was found.[20]

In his summary of the middle ear disease problem among Alaska natives and American Indians, Deuschle[3] concludes that "the most obvious common denominator for high rates of middle ear disease is a

TABLE 3 History of Draining Ear in Alaskan and Non-Alaskan Populations

Sample	Race	N	% Draining Ear More Than Once
Wasilla, Alaska	Caucasian	103	15
Alaskan teachers' children	Caucasian	162	4
Non-Alaskan teachers' children	Caucasian	99	5
St. Paul, Pribilof Islands	Aleut	95	5
7 Eskimo villages	Eskimo	1,003	23

poverty-related factor." Investigators concerned with middle ear pathology and its sequelae in Alaska concur with Deuschle in isolating socioeconomic variables as important predisposing factors influencing morbidity rates and severity.[25, 26, 39, 44] The average Eskimo household in southeastern Alaska, with its inadequate heating arrangement, poor sanitary facilities, and severe overcrowding, dramatically illustrates a high-risk environment for acute and chronic infections of all types. It is especially conducive to cross infection of upper respiratory tract disorders. Similar correlations between high rates of acute middle ear disease and poor socioeconomic conditions have been suggested by researchers studying this morbidity condition among American Indians.[29, 31, 40]

Significantly, the dramatic intervillage[43] and intertribe[30] variations in morbidity experience among Eskimos and Indians have been explained in terms of differences in socioeconomic factors. Using a rough socioeconomic index based on housing conditions, housekeeping habits, income, and family functioning, Cambon *et al.*[29] find a strong correlation between aural disease and social pathology in an Indian village, with the class rated "poor" experiencing almost six times the rate of disease found in the class rated "good." In Alaska[44] an inverse rela-

TABLE 4 Hearing Loss in Various Alaskan Populations

Sample	Race	N	Severe Loss[a] (%)
Wasilla, Alaska	Caucasian	244	1
St. Paul, Pribilof Islands	Aleut	87	1
Eskimo villages	Eskimo	327	13

[a]Loss of 40 db or more from 1,000 to 3,000 Hz, ISO 1964.

tionship between adequacy of housing, diet, and income and level of morbidity (presence of abnormal tympanic membrane) is also indicated. A more recent study,[27] however, fails to demonstrate any relationship between incidence of disease among Eskimo children and such factors as crowded living conditions and welfare status.

Significantly, other poverty groups of contrasting racial characteristics also experience high morbidity rates. The observed prevalence rates of middle ear disease and hearing loss in an economically depressed county in Appalachia[45] are given in Table 5.

Fay's recent study[19] of middle ear disease (both suppurative and nonsuppurative) among a New York ghetto population, aged 2 through 16, produces similarly striking figures. Twenty percent of 225 children given otologic examinations exhibit some form of middle ear pathology. Of the children who are given pure tone audiometric testing, nearly 20 percent are found to suffer a hearing handicap (15 db or more in one tone, ASA 1951) after correction for false positives; of the otoscopically abnormal children, 52 percent fail the screening test.

Regardless of differences in such factors as screening standards and sample framework in the above-mentioned studies, it is apparent that these groups suffer a considerable high risk of infection. Importantly, their common denominator, as Deuschle[3] suggests, is poverty and *not* race. This relationship is, however, very complex, and there is some question as to whether incidence of acute and prevalence of chronic

TABLE 5   Prevalence of Otitis Media and Hearing Loss in Martin County, Kentucky

Age Group	Total No. of Exams	Condition	Prevalence Rate (%)
0–1	220	Disorders of ear	33.6
		Acute otitis media[a]	20.0
		Chronic otitis media[a]	5.4
2–12	632	Disorders of ear	34.8
		Acute otitis media[a]	12.5
		Chronic otitis media[a]	4.1
		Hearing loss[a]	9.4
Adult	1,116	Disorders of ear	25.8
		Hearing loss[a]	23.9

[a]Diagnostic criteria not recorded.

disease should not be assessed independently for their variation by social class.

In Alaska intensive medical treatment campaigns and efforts to improve general socioeconomic conditions in selected subgroups of Eskimos yield significant reduction in the level of chronic disease* in one campaign and in the severity and duration of episodes of draining ear in another.[46] Neither, however, is able to effect significant reductions in monthly incidence of acute attacks.

Studies of general practice records in Great Britain[12,15] fail to document a significant social class gradient in incidence rates. Other investigators have found that "discharging ears" snow little relationship to social class.[47] While a report published in 1960[48] indicates that children with chronic discharge commonly come from economically deprived families, other investigators have challenged this assertion. Rein,[49] in a recent article on the National Health Service, cites an outcome study of acute middle ear infections that indicates present high quality of care delivered to lower social groups. This investigation of school-age children fails to find a relationship between drum scarring (sign of neglected acute infections) and social class. This indicates that if incidence of acute attacks is higher in lower social classes, at least care is of the quality necessary to eliminate differentials in severity by social class. Rein's provocative paper clearly emphasizes the need to delineate the relative roles of medical care and environmental/socioeconomic factors in determining morbidity levels.

Two studies conducted on urban (primarily) Caucasian populations and attempting to assess morbidity rates by social class remain to be mentioned. Findings from a morbidity survey conducted in Essex County, Canada,[50] on a population sampled from the roster of a prepaid medical care program suggest a trend of increasing rates of disease with declining socioeconomic status (Table 6). The gradient is not dramatic, but it is of interest in light of the narrow range of socioeconomic status involved; i.e., all were enrollees in a prepaid medical care plan.

A survey of Vancouver elementary school children[20] is the only study found documenting rates of serous otitis media by social class, and no direct relationship is established in that study. Significantly, the disproportionately higher rate of hearing loss observed among children with lower socioeconomic backgrounds is attributed to the

---

* J. K. Fleshman, personal communication, March 1969.

TABLE 6   Children, Age 1–19, with Otitis Media

Socioeconomic Status	Age-Standardized Proportion of Cases
upper	0.18
middle	0.17
lower	0.26

likelihood of more suppurative infections in this population. If there are contrasting patterns for serous and acute otitis media, designed epidemiologic studies might clarify the relationships.

The sibling factor remains to be mentioned. In a study of Guamanian school children,[37] a correlation is found between the number of older siblings and the likelihood of a severe hearing loss or a perforation: Perforations are seven times as common among children with five or more older siblings when compared with only children. Similar correlations between morbidity and number of siblings have been found by other investigators, although Reed and Dunn's study[27] fails to corroborate this relationship.

On the basis of the available evidence, it appears that populations with striking contrasts in socioeconomic status will exhibit parallel contrasts in severity and/or prevalence of suppurative middle ear disease. These differences may be attributable to a combination of high-risk environmental conditions and difficulty in access to medical care.

SEASONAL VARIATION

A fairly consistent pattern of seasonal variation in the incidence of otitis media has been reported in diverse populations located in contrasting geographic areas. The consensus of these reports documents peak monthly rates in the winter and early spring months with a low in mid-summer.

British studies[11, 12, 13] of acute otitis media in general practice document comparable patterns with the highest monthly rates in January through March and the lowest in July through August. Similar patterns are seen in Mississippi,[51] Baltimore,* and South Carolina.[14] Data recording the number of new cases of acute middle ear infection among Indians (excluding Alaska)[52] document a similar seasonal variation,

* R. H. Drachman, personal communication, November 1969.

with one third of the total annual cases occurring in the period December–February and winter rates twice the monthly rate recorded in summer (June–September). In Alaska investigations on the epidemiologic patterns of acute otitis media among Eskimo populations have failed to reveal a consistent seasonal variation in incidence.[24, 27] One study[24] explores the relationship between morbidity rates and temperature and wind speed; no significant correlations are discovered.

A consideration of the etiology of serous as opposed to acute purulent middle ear disease tends to lead to the assumption that different seasonal patterns exist. Evidence in the literature belies this assumption. Consider Figures 1 and 2, which trace monthly incidence levels: Although not strictly comparable, the graphs are strikingly similar. A comparison of an Alaska study of acute otitis media among Caucasians[16] and Lemon's findings[10] on serous otitis media yields similar results: Both documented peak incidence rates in March, dropping to a mid-

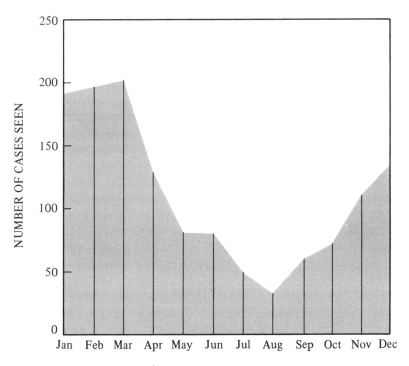

FIGURE 1   Monthly incidence pattern of acute otitis media. From Medical Research Council.[11]

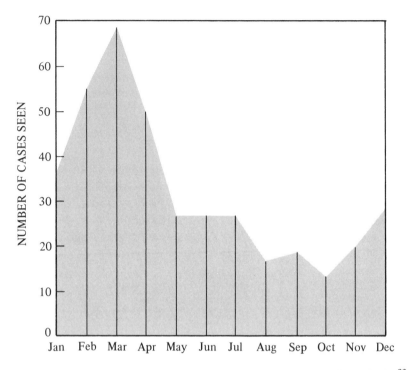

FIGURE 2 Monthly incidence pattern for serous otitis media. From Suehs.[33]

summer low (August) with December rates considerably lower than those found in the spring months.

The effects of geography and climate certainly bear more investigation. Suehs[33] has suggested that high humidity and low altitude are related to high incidence of both upper respiratory and middle ear infections (including serous), but no studies on these climatic factors were uncovered. There is fairly widespread agreement that periods of variable weather rather than general temperature levels are predisposing environmental factors in the development of middle ear infection.[12, 33]

FUNCTIONAL IMPACT

Serious complications of middle ear infections, such as mastoiditis and labyrinthitis, have become increasingly rare with the widespread use of antibiotics.[11, 34, 53] However, hearing losses in children resulting from recurrent or chronic infections of the middle ear are still a problem of significant scope.[17, 20, 33, 34, 54, 55] Investigations of the etiology of hearing loss reveal that together suppurative and nonsuppurative middle ear infections are probably responsible for well over 50 percent of all cases of hearing loss (including sensorineural) in children.[56-59]

Unfortunately, the incidence, prevalence, and severity of this disease in the general pediatric population of the United States are difficult to estimate accurately at present. (See the section on Epidemiology.) Data from Great Britain, however, indicate that approximately 50 percent of the population experience at least one attack of acute suppurative otitis media by age 8, and that as many as 17 percent may still suffer appreciable hearing losses 5 to 10 years after an acute attack.[12, 13] The incidence of nonsuppurative otitis media (serous otitis media) and its sequelae is even more difficult to appraise because it is often asymptomatic. Yet, the disease is viewed by many as the most prevalent cause of conductive hearing losses in children.[17, 20, 33, 55, 57, 58]

The focus of the present review is the impact of hearing loss secondary to middle ear infections on the general well-being and normal development of affected children. The data strongly suggest that educators have long been aware of the serious implications of severe permanent hearing loss in young children. However, contrary to popular opinion and prevailing practice, even mild to moderate (fluctuating) conductive losses (characteristic sequelae of otitis media) also may seriously impair the educational and social prognosis of affected children. It will become apparent in the course of the discussion that such information has important implications for current practice in public health, medicine, and education—not only in regard to procedures needed for the identification of affected children, but also in provisions for their medical and educational management.

PROBLEMS IN ASSESSING IMPACT

The potential consequences of hearing loss on a child's normal development are difficult to define and assess. Lack of appropriate criteria for "retardation" is one problem; for example, investigators concerned with hearing loss in children are hampered by the lack of a model representing "normal" personality development with which to assess psychosocial impact of impairment.[60] A related problem is the use of appropriate tools to measure the impact of a particular outcome of hearing loss. A blatant example of inappropriate methods would be to rely on verbal instructions to performance tests for hearing-impaired children; the literature abounds with examples less blatant, but similarly invalid. A further difficulty is the lack of determination as to what level *and duration* of impairment, as well as ear involvement, constitute an educational and social handicap, or will result in retardation. Table 7 represents an attempt to relate level of bilateral loss to educational needs. It is now recognized that such specifications are imprecise guidelines and that the educational and social prognosis of affected children is the product of an individual adjustment based on such variable factors as age of onset of impairment, degree of loss, general intelligence, emotional stability, timing and effectiveness of treatment, and educational favorability of the home.[62-65] This knowledge renders definitive statements on the functional impact of middle ear disease difficult; for example, it is possible that among cultural subgroups of the population, such as Eskimos, prevalence of hearing loss secondary to chronic otitis media and academic retardation are less directly related than academic retardation and social factors.[27,66] It becomes clear that the reputed causal relationship between hearing loss and educational and social adjustment is subject to many intervening factors that are difficult to control in a study situation.

Although much work has been done on the habilitation and rehabilitation of children with severe sensorineural hearing impairment, there are few studies that directly assess the impact of hearing loss associated with otitis media. Research is lacking on preschool children with moderate hearing impairments, and investigations on similarly handicapped school-age children seldom analyze measures of academic performance by type of impairment (i.e., sensorineural versus conductive). Although the literature is sparse in the area of psychosocial adjustment to hearing loss, it consistently points to the apparent relationship between minimal hearing loss and educational and social maladjustment.

IMPACT ON EDUCATION PROGRESS

Early Work   The dominant area of inquiry concerning children with hearing impairment has been the assessment of impact by measures of academic performance and achievement. As early as 1935 it was noted that hearing loss is approximately 15 times more prevalent among children retarded in reading than in those with average or better reading skills.[67] Similarly, a decade later Schonell and Schonell[68] find that among children retarded in spelling, 6.7 percent had "defective" hearing versus 4.5 percent of control children judged good in spelling. A later study by Burt[69] reveals that among children with normal educational attainments, 1 percent exhibit a marked hearing loss and 4 percent a slight impairment, whereas those considered "backward" by the same measures have a prevalence of 6 and 12–18 percent respectively. Waldon[70] subsequently reports finding significant differences between normal children and a combined group of deaf and hard-of-hearing children on measures of sentence length and type. In a review of the literature up to 1957, Young and McConnell[71] conclude that hearing-impaired children are usually "retarded" ½–2 years in school and lack normal language ability.

Recent Work   Using achievement test scores, Kodman[72] attempts to assess the influence of mild to moderate hearing loss on educational achievement in a normal school environment. One hundred Kentucky public school children between the ages of 7 and 17 with an IQ of 80–120 and mild to moderate hearing losses (speech reception threshold 20–65 db) were administered a standardized test to measure grade achievement. Results demonstrate that on the average this hearing-impaired group is not only achieving below their actual grade placement (grade 3.84 as opposed to 4.84), but far below their normal grade level (6.08).

Instead of using a standardized test, Wishik *et al.*[73] measure academic retardation with grade repetition rate, actual grade placement, and age of admission to school. When audiometric test scores, taken from 1946 to 1954, for over a thousand children aged 5–14 are analyzed, it is determined that only 5.9 percent of the children admitted at the normal age have ever failed an audiometric test as opposed to 11.5 percent of those admitted late. Moreover, children who have ever failed an audiometric test during their school career are twice as likely to repeat an academic grade as other children. The audiometric failure rate among those children 2 years behind is found to be far greater than for those children only 1 year behind and three times as high as the rate among children in the normal grade. The observed grade–age relationship also delineates sharp differences: Among 114 children ever failing an audiometric exam, nearly 40 percent have not reached their normal academic level at the end of the study versus 25 percent of those children never failing the tests. Significant to the present discussion is the suggestion by Wishik *et al.*[73] that a child need not have a severe permanent loss to experience problems in school. Rather, even a single failure on an audiometric test over his entire school career—such as would be caused by a mild temporary hearing

TABLE 7 Relationship of Degree of Handicap to Educational Needs

Degree of Handicap	Effect of Hearing Loss on the Understanding of Language and Speech	Educational Needs and Programs
Slight 16–29 db (ASA) or 27–40 db (ISO)	May have difficulty hearing faint or distant speech. Will not usually experience difficulty in school situations.	May benefit from a hearing aid as loss approaches 30db (ASA) or 40db (ISO). Attention to vocabulary development. Needs favorable seating and lighting. May need lip reading instruction. May need speech correction.
Mild 30–44 db (ASA) or 41–55 db (ISO)	Understands conversational speech at a distance of 3–5 feet (face-to-face). May miss as much as 50 percent of class discussions if voices are faint or not in line of vision. May exhibit limited vocabulary and speech anomalies.	Child should be referred to special education for educational follow-up if such service is available. Individual hearing aid by evaluation and training in its use. Favorable seating and possible special class placement, especially for primary children. Attention to vocabulary and reading. May need lip reading instruction. Speech conservation and correction, if indicated.
Marked 45–59 db (ASA) or 56–70 db (ISO)	Conversation must be loud to be understood. Will have increasing difficulty with school situations requiring participation in group discussions. Is likely to have defective speech. Is likely to be deficient in language usage and comprehension.	Will need resource teacher or special class. Special help in language skills, vocabulary development, usage, reading, writing, grammar, etc. Individual hearing aid by evaluation and auditory training.

52

Class and hearing level	Ability to hear / speech and language	Educational needs
(continued from previous page)	Will have evidence of limited vocabulary.	Lip reading instruction. Speech conservation and speech correction. Attention to auditory and visual situations at all times.
Severe 60–79 db (ASA) or 71–90 db (ISO)	May hear loud voices about one foot from the ear. May be able to identify environmental sounds. May be able to discriminate vowels but not all consonants. Speech and language defective and likely to deteriorate. Speech and language will not develop spontaneously if loss is present before one year of age.	Will need full-time special program for deaf children, with emphasis on all language skills, concept development, lip reading, and speech. Program needs specialized supervision and comprehensive supporting services. Individual hearing aid by evaluation. Auditory training on individual and group aids. Part-time in regular classes only as profitable.
Extreme 80 db or more (ASA) or 91 db or more (ISO)	May hear some loud sounds but is aware of vibrations more than tonal pattern. Relies on vision rather than hearing as primary avenue for communication. Speech and language defective and likely to deteriorate. Speech and language will not develop spontaneously if loss is present before one year.	Will need full-time in special program for deaf children, with emphasis on all language skills, concept development, lip reading, and speech. Program needs specialized supervision and comprehensive supporting services. Continuous appraisal of needs in regard to oral and manual communication. Auditory training on group and individual aid. Part-time in regular classes only for carefully selected children.

Source: Bernero and Bothwell.[66]

53

loss following an infection of the middle ear—appears to place him at higher risk of experiencing academic retardation.

Since measurements of grade level achievement are at best gross criteria for retardation and often inappropriate tools for meaningfully assessing impact of hearing loss, investigators often study specific language skills in this connection. An example is the study conducted by Young and McConnell[71] designed to investigate whether the vocabulary level of hearing-impaired children enrolled in regular classes differs significantly from that of normal hearing children of similar age, race, sex, nonverbal intelligence, and socioeconomic level.

The children chosen for the experimental group (N=20) were white, between the ages of 8 and 14, had all developed basic oral language skills without the aid of special instruction, and recorded average hearing losses in the better ear of 30 db or more (500–2,000 Hz, ASA). Mean hearing loss was 51 db, and individual levels ranged from 32 to 75 db. A control group of normal-hearing children (N=20) was matched for age, race, sex, socioeconomic background (using factors such as type of neighborhood, education, and income level of parents), and nonverbal intelligence (as measured by Raven's Progressive Matrices, a test not dependent on oral or written instructions for completion).

Both groups were administered the Ammons Full-Range Picture Vocabulary Test, which is designed to allow optimal performance independent of reading ability and verbal fluency. Results reveal highly significant differences between the hearing-impaired and normal-hearing children (Table 8). It is evident that "even a mild to moderate hearing loss in children is apt to result in retarded language functioning"[71]; not one hearing-impaired child scored higher than his matched control.

Noteworthy in this study is the fact that the authors recognize socioeconomic and intelligence variables, as well as past correction status, to be of potential significance in determining both educational impact of hearing loss and test performance in general. Moreover, their measurement tool, which separated vocabulary skills from verbal fluency and reading ability, was aptly chosen. Unfortunately for our purposes, information is again lacking on the relationship of age of onset and kind of impairment to language skills. However, the degree of loss in the speech frequencies experienced by the sample children is roughly comparable to that which can occur secondary to bilateral chronic otitis media. In view of these shortcomings, Ling's study[74] merits attention.

TABLE 8 Summary of *t* Scores Comparing Mean Vocabulary Test Raw Scores of 20 Matched Pairs of Hearing-Impaired and Normal-Hearing Children

Group	Mean Raw Score Vocabulary Test	Difference	*t* Score[a]
Hard of hearing	31.45		
		17.75	6.72
Normal hearing	49.20		

[a]A *t* score of 2.093 is required for significance at 0.05 confidence level, and 2.861 is required for significance at 0.01 confidence level.
Source: Young and McConnell.[71]

His study group consisted of all children with known hearing defects attending normal schools in Reading, Scotland, in 1956 (*N*= 42, 39 cooperating); severity of deafness ranged from less than 15 db to more than 60 db, ASA. The survey design consisted of assessments of hearing (pure tone and speech audiometry), speech, educational attainments (Schonell's Diagnostic and Attainment Tests; Reading Test R1, R3; Essential Mechanical and Essential Problem Arithmetic Tests), mental ability (Stanford-Binet), and social background (parent's occupation plus Sommer's rating system of home environment). In addition, medical history data were obtained (Table 9). As seen in Table 9, the large majority of these children have mild or moderate losses. Yet the results of the achievement tests indicate that with one exception children are retarded in either reading or arithmetic

TABLE 9 Distribution of Hearing Defects in Terms of Severity as Measured by Pure Tones and Speech Audiometry

Method of Measurement	Distribution of Hearing Defects			
Pure tone				
Hearing loss[a]	<25 db	25–40 db	40–60 db	>60 db
No. children	21	10	7	1
Speech audiometry				
Discrimination[b]	0	0–10%	10–40%	>40%
No. children	8	13	15	3

[a]Average over 5 tones, 500–4,000 Hz, ASA.
[b]Average percent failure at 55, 70, and 85 db.
Source: Adapted from Ling.[74]

or both. These findings are highly significant since it is also found that the group is skewed toward greater than average intelligence as measured by three tests. Of great importance are the findings that (a) degree of retardation was positively associated with degree of impairment, and (b) children with slight losses as measured by pure tones and no significant discrimination problems also showed a significant degree of backwardness (Table 10). These findings are recently confirmed in Quigley's[62] study of Illinois public school children with mild to moderate hearing impairments, in which it is demonstrated that impairments significantly less than 26 db ISO in the better ear are also apparently related to academic progress (Table 11).

Analysis of the kind of hearing loss in Ling's series reveals only 7 sensorineural cases out of 39 total. Medical records show that at least 28 children had received treatment for ear, nose, and throat problems over periods ranging from a few months to 10 years. Significantly, audiograms recorded on these children show considerable variability in hearing levels (a finding confirmed by parents) and primarily associated with colds, clearly indicating middle ear involvement. Although no precise information is available on age of onset, many parents recognized hearing loss in their children at age 3. This finding of common preschool involvement may partially explain the fact that much of the

TABLE 10   Average Retardation, in Months, on Four Achievement Tests in Terms of Severity of Defect as Measured by Pure Tones and Speech Audiometry

Pure Tone				
Hearing loss (db, ASA)	<25	25–40	40–60	>60
No. children	21	10	7	1
Test R 1	16	20	27	–
Test R 3	9	11	19	–
Problem arithmetic	14	25	35	16
Mechanical arithmetic	14	23	29	9
Speech Audiometry				
Discrimination loss (%)	0	<40	>40	
No. children	8	28	3	
Test R 1	16	18	41	
Test R 3	10	8	43	
Problem arithmetic	15	20	41	
Mechanical arithmetic	14	19	41	

Source: Adapted from Ling.[74]

TABLE 11   Differences Between Expected Performance and Actual Performance of the Subjects on Various Subtests of the Stanford Achievement Test

Hearing Threshold Level in Better Ear (db, ISO)	N	IQ	Word Meaning	Paragraph Meaning	Language	Subtest Average
<15	59	105.14	−1.04	−0.47	−0.78	−0.73
15–26	37	100.81	−1.40	−0.86	−1.16	−1.11
27–40	6	103.50	−3.48	−1.78	−1.95	−2.31
41–55	9	97.89	−3.84	−2.54	−2.93	−3.08
56–70	5	92.40	−2.78	−2.20	−3.52	−2.87
TOTAL	116[a]	102.56	−1.66	−0.90	−1.30	−1.25

[a]Expected grade placement in school (N=116): Mean, 690; SD, 2.63.
  Actual grade placement in school (N=116): Mean, 5.78; SD, 2.61.
Source: Quigley.[62]

academic retardation experienced apparently occurs during the first 3 years of schooling.

Other findings of interest in Ling's study follow: Of the 39 affected children, 22 have speech defects; presence of speech defects is inversely related to social class, while average retardation varies little between social groups (occupation) or in relation to home rating scores; the proportion of cases with conductive deafness is greater among children in the lower social groups. Unfortunately, while utilization of hearing aids is mentioned, no attempt is made to relate use to academic achievement.

The lack of a control group in this study renders certain assumptions necessary. The most important is that the norms published for the educational tests used are valid for Reading school children.* Yet the importance of Ling's study in assessing the needs of the hearing-impaired child in the normal classroom is emphasized in a consideration of Scottish criteria for "significant deafness" in operation at the time: Any child with hearing better than 35 db in the better ear is judged capable of full benefit from normal education "without change or addition."† Ling's finding of significant retardation in children with even

---

* Quigley's study[62] suffers the same shortcomings from lack of a control group; he assumes test validity on the basis of the fact that his study population came from an upper socioeconomic group (Table 11).
† Similarly, no special educational provisions had been made for *any* child in Quigley's series.

mild losses clearly appears to challenge these earlier norms. No clear explanation for this discovery is apparent; the author hypothesizes that perhaps adverse noise conditions would bother these children more than those with normal hearing, or that possibly an earlier and more severe conductive loss since treated had left these children with a residual educational handicap.

Aware of the methodologic problems that render his study inconclusive though highly suggestive, Ling designed a second survey[66] to test whether the relationship between hearing loss secondary to otitis media and academic retardation was, in fact, causal. Children with a history of otitis media attending regular classes and with hearing losses at the time of the study ranging from 15 to 45 db A S A were matched with children from the "same background, controlling for home environment, school attendance, intelligence and social maturity." Results from administration of Schonell's achievement tests reveal that by 9–10 years of age the hearing-impaired group was retarded in problem arithmetic by 19 months in relation to controls, in mechanical arithmetic by 16 months, and in mechanical reading by 15 months. As found in Ling's earlier study,[74] degree of retardation is positively related to severity of hearing loss, although children with mildest losses again evince significant academic handicaps. Moreover, follow-up of younger hearing-impaired children reveals that retardation occurring early in a child's school career[5, 17, 20, 54] is not generally overcome without remedial teaching.

While Ling's study[66] merely implicates otitis media as the causative factor in academic retardation on the basis of medical history items, Holm and Kunze[75] directly assess educational impact of hearing losses accompanying currently diagnosed cases of chronic otitis media. Cases and controls were selected from the population of an outpatient department on the basis of the following criteria: All were between the ages of 5 and 9; all attended regular classes and had normal attendance records; and no child exhibited obvious mental retardation, related signs, or congenital anomalies. The children had no chronic conditions other than otitis media, had all experienced onset of middle ear pathology before 2 years of age, had pathology in both ears (bilateral), and had been characterized by fluctuating hearing acuity as observed by parents and recorded in the ear, nose, and throat clinic. Hearing loss at the time of testing was judged not severe enough to interfere with language tests used in the study. Controls, matched for age, sex, race, and socioeconomic level, had no chronic conditions, no documented episodes of middle ear infection, and normal tympanic membranes and hearing acuity at the time of the survey.

Both groups of children were given a battery of tests designed to measure language and speech development. Results are described in Figure 3. As measured by these tests, the experimental group was delayed to a significant degree in all language skills requiring the reception and processing of auditory stimuli or the production of verbal responses, i.e., the acquisition of vocabulary skills, ability to receive and express ideas through spoken language, the use of grammar and syntax, and auditory memory skills. No significant differences are found in tests measuring primarily visual and motor skills. Although these findings are very impressive, extrapolation to other population groups is not completely justified. While overcoming many shortcomings found in earlier investigations, such as generally careful matching of cases and controls, attention to age of onset, potentially significant concomitant health problems and school attendance patterns, the size of the sample was very small. Also, the significance of possible differences in mental ability between groups was not considered, and valuable analyses, such as test performance in relation to treatment and actual academic progress, not undertaken.

IMPACT ON PSYCHOSOCIAL ADJUSTMENT

Relatively little work has been done relating psychosocial adjustment and hearing impairment in children. Perhaps one of the reasons is the difficulty in designing procedures and determining criteria for assessing social "abnormality" or "retardation." Only three studies were found that attempted to study these factors in children with mild to moderate hearing losses.

In Ling's study,[74] all children were administered the Vineland Social Maturity Scale. In addition, teachers' ratings on six personality factors were obtained. Analysis of results fails to reveal a clear trend toward social retardation as measured by the Vineland Scale. Children were judged by teachers above average in disposition and behavior, while below average in concentration, initiative, and self-confidence. The small sample size and subjectiveness of the ratings prevent generalizations.

A more definitive study was undertaken by Fisher,[56] one of the few investigators who addresses himself directly to the issue of whether mild to moderate hearing losses are of any real consequence in re-

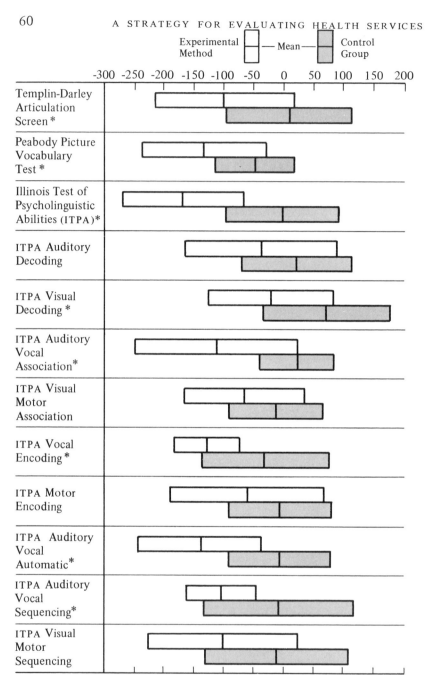

FIGURE 3   Standard score means and standard deviations for the experimental and control groups on tests administered to children. From Holm and Kunze.[75] Asterisk designates tests for which group differences are significant at 0.05 level of confidence.

gard to the emotional and social adjustment of affected children. His study group consisted of public school children who had been kept under regular audiologic review because of chronic hearing problems (*N*=82); at the time of the investigation ages ranged from 5.4 to 16.0 years and hearing losses from 20 to 64 db British Standard (BS) with a mean of 38 db. A control group was assembled systematically by selecting the next child of the same sex on the class register. Both groups were administered the widely used Bristol Social Adjustment Guide. When mean scores for both are compared, a statistically significant difference is revealed, with 47 percent of the hearing-impaired children and 28 percent of the controls judged abnormally adjusted as measured by this scale. Analysis of the type of maladjustment (Bristol Guide syndromes) among the hearing-impaired group reveals that, contrary to expectations, there is more demonstrative and mixed behavior than withdrawing behavior. Four factors are found to be associated with the adjustment of these children: nonverbal ability, chronological age, educational favorability of the home, and all-around school progress. (As a group, the hearing-impaired children show significant retardation in the basic subjects.) Children over 11 show the best adjustment, and those 5–8 have a lower rate of maladjustment than children 8–11; also, girls exhibit more marked differences in amount and type of maladjustment than do boys when compared to the nor-normal-hearing group. Explanations for these findings are not readily apparent. Significantly, Fisher finds no association between degree of loss, or type of loss, and degree of maladjustment. These results do imply that hearing problems in the ordinary classroom, though not severe, are associated with concomitant emotional and social maladjustment. As Fisher notes, "Impaired hearing, poor adjustment and scholastic failure may interact to produce retardation out of all proportion to the degree of hearing loss."

A related inquiry is represented by Gilles' study,[76] in which conclusions on cognitive development and psychosocial adjustment of hearing-impaired children were approached by studying patterns of differences between their drawings of "a person" and "myself" and those of normal-hearing children. A combined group of deaf and partially hearing children between the ages of 5 and 15, attending both special and public schools in the Glasgow, Scotland, area, were matched by age and sex with children in public schools in the area. The sets of drawings obtained from each child were scored on the scale of the Goodenough Draw-a-Man Test. Consistent patterns of qualitative differences emerge between the groups (none between the deaf and hard-of-hearing groups). The drawings of "self" among the hearing-impaired children tend to be much larger and richer in detail than drawings of "a person"; the reverse pattern is exhibited in normally hearing children. The author hypothesizes that such differences could be attributed to variation in cognitive development (e.g., body-image distortion), psychosocial adjustment, or such factors as differential practice or fatigue. While controls are rudimentary and criteria "somewhat arbitrarily adopted," this study represents an interesting approach in a neglected area concerning impact of hearing loss in children.

REFERENCES

1. Mawson SR: Diseases of the Middle Ear. London, Edward Arnold, Ltd, 1963
2. Shambeaugh GE Jr: Surgery of the Ear. Philadelphia, WB Saunders Co, 1959
3. Deuschle KW: A report on the middle ear disease problem among the American Indian and Alaska natives (mimeographed report). New York, Department of Community Medicine, Mt. Sinai School of Medicine, March 1969.
4. Suehs OW: Secretory otitis media. Laryngoscope 62:998–1027, 1952
5. Campbell EH: The prevention of deafness in acute infections of the middle ear. Pa Med J 57:1173–1178, 1954
6. Nielson JC: Studies of the Aetiology of Acute Otitis Media. Copenhagen, Ejnar Munkegasrd, 1945.
7. Feingold M, Klein JO, Haslan GE, et al: Acute otitis media in children. Am J Dis Child 3:361–365, 1966
8. Fernandez AA, McGovern JP: Secretory otitis media in allergic infants and children. South Med J 58:581–585, 1965
9. Yunginger J: Cited by Chan JCM, Logan GB, and McBean JB: Serous otitis media and allergy. Am J Dis Child 114:684–692, 1967
10. Lemon AN: Serous otitis media in children. Laryngoscope 72:32–44, 1962
11. Medical Research Council: Acute otitis media in general practice. Lancet 2:510–514, 1957
12. Fry J, Dillane JB, Jones RF, et al: The outcome of acute otitis media Br J Prev Soc Med 23:205–209, 1969
13. Lowe JF, Bamforth JS, Pracy R: Acute otitis media: One year in a general practice. Lancet 2:1129–1132, 1963
14. Brownlee RG, Delouche WR, Cowan CC, et al: Otitis media in children. Pediatrics 75:636–642, 1966
15. Logan WPD: Morbidity Statistics from General Practice. London, HM Stationery Office, 1960

16. Reed D, Brody J: Otitis media in urban Alaska. Alaska Med 8:64–67, 1966
17. Armstrong BW: Chronic secretory otitis media: Diagnosis and treatment. South Med J 50:540–546, 1957
18. Jordon R: Chronic secretory otitis media. Laryngoscope 59:1002–1015, 1949
19. Fay TH, Hochberg I, Smith CR, et al: Audiologic and otologic screening of disadvantaged children. Arch Otolaryngol 91:366–368, 1970
20. Robinson GC, Anderson DO, Moghadam HK, et al: A survey of hearing loss in Vancouver school children. I. Methodology and prevalence. Can Med Assoc J 97:1199–1207, 1967
21. Eagles EL, Wishik SM, Doefler LG: Hearing sensitivity and ear disease in children: A prospective study. Laryngoscope, Monograph Suppl., 1967
22. Eagles EL, Wishik SM, Doefler LG, et al: Hearing sensitivity and related factors in children. Laryngoscope, Monograph Suppl., 1963
23. Brody JA: Notes on the epidemiology of draining ears and hearing loss in Alaska with comments on future studies and control measures. Alaska Med 6:1–4, 1964
24. Maynard JE: Otitis media in Alaska Eskimo children: An epidemiologic review with observations on control. Alaska Med:93–97, 1969
25. Reed D, Struve S, Maynard JE: Otitis media and hearing deficiency among Eskimo children: A cohort study. Am J Public Health 57:1657–1662, 1967
26. Ling D, McCoy RH, Levinson ED: The incidence of middle ear disease and its educational implications among Baffin Island Eskimo children. Am J Public Health 60:385–390, 1969
27. Reed D, Dunn W: Epidemiologic studies of otitis media among Eskimo children. Public Health Rep 85:699–707, 1970
28. Dolowitz DA: Hearing rehabilitation with modified radical mastoidectomy. Tex State Med J 59:962–967, 1963
29. Cambon K, Galbraith JD, Kong G: Middle ear disease in Indians of the Mount Currie Reservation, British Columbia. Can Med Assoc J 93:1301–1305, 1965
30. Zonis RD: Chronic otitis media in the southwestern American Indian. I. Prevalence. Arch Otolaryngol 88:360–365, 1968
31. Gregg JB, Steele JP, Clifford S, Werthman HG: A multidisciplinary study of ear disease in South Dakota Indian children. SD J Med 23:11–20, 1970
32. Jaffee BF: The incidence of ear diseases in the Navajo Indian. Laryngoscope 79:2126–2134, 1969
33. Suehs OW: Secretory otitis media. Laryngoscope 62:998–1027, 1952
34. Fry J, Jones REMc, Kalton G, et al: The outcome of acute otitis media. Br J Prev Soc Med 23:205–209, 1969
35. Beaver R: Defective hearing in children attending ordinary schools. J R Inst Public Health 28:119–127, 1965
36. Bjuggren G, Tunevall G: Otitis in childhood. Acta Otolaryngol 45:311–328, 1952
37. Eldridge R, Brody JA, Wetmore N: Hearing loss and otitis media on Guam. Arch Otolaryngol 91:148–153, 1970

38. Tetrakis NL, Molohan KT, Tepper DJ: Cerumen in American Indians: Genetic implications of the sticky and dry types. Science 158:1192–1193, 1967

39. Otitis Media Planning Committee: Program plan for otitis media (mimeographed report). Anchorage, Alaska Division of Public Health, 1968

40. Johnson RL: Chronic otitis media in school age Navajo Indians. Laryngoscope 78:1990–1995, 1967

41. Jaffee BF, Hurtado F, and Hurtado E: Tympanic membrane mobility in the newborn. Laryngoscope 80:36–48, 1968

42. Public Health Service: Indian Health Trends and Services, 1969, Washington, DC, Government Printing Office, 1969

43. Brody JA, Overfield T, McAlister R: Draining ears and deafness among Alaska Eskimos. Arch Otolaryngol 81:29–33, 1965

44. Hayman CR, Kester FE: EENT infections in natives of Alaska. Northwest Med 56:423–430, 1957

45. Health status of the population of Martin County, Kentucky, 1964-1965 (mimeographed report). Lexington, Department Community Medicine, University of Kentucky, January 1966

46. Maynard JE: Otitis media conference report and recommendations (mimeographed report). Anchorage, Epidemiology Section, Alaska Division of Public Health, December 1967

47. Douglas JWB, Blomfield JM: Children under Five. London, Allen and Unwin, 1958

48. Miller FJW: Growing Up in Newcastle-upon-Tyne. London, Oxford University Press, 1960

49. Rein M: Social class and the utilization of medical care services. Hospitals 43:43–54, 1969

50. Laughton KB, Buck CW, Hobbs GE: Socioeconomic status and illness. Milbank Mem Fund Q 36:46–57, 1958

51. Coffey JS, Marton AB: Otitis media in the practice of pediatrics. Pediatrics 38:25–32, 1958

52. Public Health Service: Indian Health Service Annual Statistical Review: Hospital and Medical Services. Washington, DC, Government Printing Office, 1969

53. Harper, PA: Preventive Pediatrics: Child Health and Development. New York, Appleton-Century-Crofts, 1962

54. Olmsted RW, Alvarez MC, Moroney JD, et al: The pattern of hearing following acute otitis media. Pediatrics 65:252–255, 1961

55. Stevens D: Serous otitis as a cause of catarrhal deafness in children. Lancet 2:22–24, 1958

56. Fisher B: The social and emotional adjustment of children with impaired hearing attending ordinary classes. Br J Educ Psychol 36:319–321, 1966

57. Sataloff J, Vassallo L: Hearing loss in children. Pediatr Clin N Am 12:895–917, 1965

58. Frederickson JM: Otitis media and its complications, 1967 and 1968. Arch Otolaryngol 90:387–393, 1969

59. Kinney CE: The school age child. Hear News 18:5–7, 1950
60. Ives LA: Development of personality–emotional–social adjustment in deaf and partially hearing children. Public Health (London) 83:78–88, 1969
61. Bernero RJ, Bothwell H: Relationship of hearing impairment to educational needs. Springfield, Illinois Department of Public Health and Office of the Superintendent of Public Instruction, 1966
62. Quigley SP: Some effects of hearing impairment upon school performance. (mimeographed manuscript prepared for the Division of Special Education Services, Office of the Superintendent of Public Instruction for the State of Illinois). Springfield, 1970
63. Eagles EL, Hardy WG, Catlin FI: Human Communication: The Public Health Aspects of Hearing, Language and Speech Disorders. Washington, DC, Government Printing Office, 1968
64. Johnson JC: Educating Hearing Impaired Children in Ordinary School. Washington, DC, Volta Bureau, 1962
65. Committee on Child Health: Services for Children with Hearing Impairment. New York, American Public Health Service, 1956
66. Ling D: Rehabilitation of cases with deafness secondary to otitis media. Presented at the National Otitis Media Conference, Dallas, Texas, May 1970
67. Polling HM: Auditory deficiencies in poor readers, Clinical Studies in Reading. Supplementary Educational Monograph. Edited by HM Robinson. Chicago, University of Chicago Press, 1953
68. Schonell FJ, Schonell FE: Backwardness in Basic Subjects. London, Oliver and Boyd, 1946
69. Burt C: The Backward Child. London, London University Press, 1950
70. Waldon EF: A study of the spoken and written language of hearing impaired children. Ohio State University (Ph.D dissertation), 1963
71. Young C, McConnell F: Retardation of vocabulary development in hard of hearing children. Except Child:368–370, 1957
72. Kodman F: Educational status of the hard of hearing children in the classroom. J Speech Hear Res 28:297–299, 1963
73. Wishik SM, Kramm ER, Koch EM: Audiometric testing of school children. Public Health Rep 73:265–278, 1958
74. Ling D: Survey of children with defective hearing attending normal schools, Annual Report of the School Medical Officer, 1955. County Borough of Reading, 1956
75. Holm VA, Kunze LH: Effect of chronic otitis media on language and speech development. Pediatrics 43:833–839, 1969
76. Gilles J: Variations in drawings of "a person" and "myself" by hearing impaired and normal children. Br J Educ Psychol 38:86–89, 1968

BIBLIOGRAPHY

AMA Council on Drugs: AMA Drug Evaluation, 1971. Chicago, American Medical Association, 1971

Baron SH: Medical Treatment of Otitis Media in Otitis Media: Proceedings of the National Conference. Edited by A Glorig, KS Gerwin. Springfield, Illinois, Charles C Thomas 1972

Stickler GB, Rubenstein MM, McBean, JB, et al: Treatment of Acute Otitis Media in Children. IV. A Fourth Clinical Trial. Am J Dis Child 114:123–130, 1967

The Medical Letter Reference Handbook. Reprints of Special Issues of The Medical Letter. New York, Drug and Therapeutic Information, Inc, 1971

THREE

Visual Disorders

SUMMARY

The value of visual disorders as a tracer condition is its use as an indicator of screening procedures. The following questions should be posed: Are children in the age group 4–11 screened for visual disorders? If so, what techniques are employed? Who carrries out the vision screening? What mechanisms exist for follow-up of those children who fail the screening tests? How does the primary physician or delivery unit refer these children?

CLASSIFICATION

It has been estimated that one fourth of the 50.7 million school children in the United States require professional visual care. These visual problems are usually detected by vision screening programs that are not diagnostic of specific disorders, but indicative of the need for further evaluation. The most prevalent disorders are refractive errors, which include hyperopia (farsightedness), myopia (nearsightedness), astigmatism, and anisometropia. Strabismus, or squint, an abnormality of the coordinated movements of the eye, is less prevalent than refractive errors. Least common are the organic eye disorders and amblyopia, with the latter most frequently secondary to strabismus and anisometropia.

EPIDEMIOLOGY

Age   The failure rate of vision screening tests ranges from 5–10 percent in the 3- to 5-year age group to 16–31 percent in adolescents 12–15 years old. In general, uncorrected (without the individual's normal lenses) visual acuity for distant objects appears to improve from age 5 to 8, but then rapidly declines; uncorrected acuity for near objects improves from age 7 until age 20. Defective distance vision is over four times as common as defective near vision in the 7–20 age group.

Sex   Boys generally have better uncorrected distance and near visual acuity than girls, and fewer boys wear corrective lenses. When considering severe impairments and blindness, boys show a prevalence rate 16 to 26 percent greater than girls. When the subjects are tested wearing their usual correction, differences by sex are essentially eliminated. Generally, the percentage of people with corrective lenses increases with age, with the proportion of females greater than the proprotion of males at all age levels.

Race   Negro children of both sexes and at all age levels have better uncorrected visual acuity than white children. However, black children have been found to have a higher prevalence rate (by nearly 20 percent) of severe impairment and blindness than white children, caused chiefly by prenatal disorders and infectious diseases. The National Health Interview Survey of 1965–1966 finds that 16 percent of the white population and 9.2 percent of the nonwhite population between ages 3 and 16 have corrective lenses. Furthermore, nonwhites obtain their corrective lenses later in life, and when tested with their usual corrective lenses, the visual acuity is substantially poorer for nonwhites than whites at all age levels and for both males and females.

Socioeconomic Status   The prevalence of uncorrected deficiencies of visual acuity among children does not appear to vary with social class, although such a relationship does become apparent in adults. There is, however, an inverse relationship between family income and the severity of visual defects in children. Further, a positive correlation exists between family income and the number of children who have corrective lenses and the adequacy of their correction. These same relationships hold for adults and even stronger associations are found between educational level attained and adequacy of correction.

Geographic Distribution   No significant differences in distribution of uncorrected acuity levels by geographic region have been found in the United States. Fewer people in the South have normal corrected vision, and more southerners report severe impairments and blindness. These findings, however, are strongly related to race. When the white population is considered alone, regional differences are essentially eliminated. Rural children tend to have slightly better uncorrected vision than urban children, but rural farm children report a higher prevalence of severe visual impairment and blindness than urban children.

Functional Impact   It has been estimated that approximately 1 in 500 of the school-age population has an uncorrectable visual problem that could interfere with learning. However, the relationship between visual function and learning is complex and difficult to define precisely. There are data from the 1940s and 1950s that purport to demonstrate that correctable refractive errors and disorders of coordinative eye movement have higher prevalence rates in children with a reading disability than in controls. Other investigators suggest that although correctable visual disorders contribute to reading disability, they are usually not a principal cause of reading failure. Recently, the complex relationships between the eye and problems of learning disability, dyslexia, and other forms of school underachievement have been reviewed by an *ad hoc* committee of the American Academy of Pediatrics, the American Academy of Ophthalmology and Otolaryngology, and the American Association of Ophthalmology. It is their considered opinion that "children with learning disabilities have the same incidence of ocular abnormalities, e.g., refractive errors and muscle imbalance, as children who are normal achievers and reading at grade level."

A PLAN FOR VISION SCREENING IN CHILDREN 4–11 YEARS OF AGE

I. History

    A. When was vision acuity last tested?
    B. Who carried out the test?
    C. Does the child wear corrective lenses?
    D. Who prescribed the lenses?
    E. Has the child with lenses been re-examined in the past year?

II. Screening (yearly for all children with or without glasses)

A. *For acuity at distance.* (1) Screening tests for ages 4–5: Snellen Single Target "E" cards at 20 feet. (Test at 10 feet if child is untestable at 20 feet.) Test for monocular acuity, with and without corrective lenses. For ages 6–11: Linear Snellen "E" chart at 20 feet. Test for monocular acuity, with and without corrective lenses. (2) Fail criteria for ages 4–7: worse than 20/40 in either eye (inability to read simple majority of 20/40 symbols). Child also referred for a two-line difference in acuity between eyes. For ages 8–11: worse than 20/30 in either eye (inability to read simple majority of 20/30 symbols). Child also referred for a two-line difference in acuity between eyes.

B. *For organic defects.* (1) Screening tests for external exam of eye with flashlight to include: lids [do not refer if symptoms obviously associated with upper respiratory infection (URI)]; globe; conjunctiva [do not refer if symptoms obviously associated with (URI)]; sclera; cornea; anterior chamber; iris and pupils lens; (2) fail criteria: any external abnormality (except that due to URI).

C. *For ocular motility.* (1) Screening tests employed: monocular cover test (cover–uncover) with distant (20 feet) and near (14 in.) accomodative targets; (2) fail criteria: any tropia—constant or intermittent.

III. Management

A. *Children who fail screening test.* Should be referred for specialty care.

B. *Children who have glasses who have not been re-examined in the previous year.* Should be referred for specialty care.

EPIDEMIOLOGY

The total number of children with visual disorders is not known. It has been estimated, however, that 20–25 percent of the 50.7 million school children in the United States require some form of professional visual care.[1-5] There is no comparable estimate for the approximately 21.7 million preschool-age children.[1-5]

The majority of pediatric visual problems are detected by vision screening programs conducted by schools and community and state clinics. Such screening procedures are not diagnostic of a specific visual disorder but indicative of the need for further evaluation. The most commonly employed screening technique is visual acuity measurement utilizing a procedure based on the Snellen method.[6,7] Defective visual acuity usually indicates refractive errors, ocular misalignment, amblyopia, and/or organic problems.

Five major epidemiological aspects—age, sex, race, socioeconomic status, and geographic location—of uncorrected and "corrected" vision* are analyzed below. In each section uncorrected visual acuity, "corrected" visual acuity and referral rates are discussed. Referral rates indicate the number of children who failed the screening test; it is assumed that these children are tested wearing their usual lenses.

AGE

At birth, the eyeball is relatively closer to its adult size than most other structures. Approximate adult size is reached between the ages of 8 and 9 years, with little growth after age 16.[6,8]

Hyperopia is the usual status of the child from the time of birth until he is approximately 6 years old. During this time the degree of hyperopia decreases as the axial length of the eye increases. Refraction approaches normal between ages 7 and 8. As the eye continues to grow, myopia may develop. This condition represents a lack of coordination between the length of the eyeball and the optical power of the cornea and lens, and its onset is often coincident with puberty. Myopia tends to increase irregularly during puberty and periods of rapid growth in the teens and usually, except in the case of "progressive myopia," stabilizes by age 20.[6,7,9-11]

Figure 1 shows the basic changes by age in the failure rate of vision screening tests for specific conditions without usual correction. An increase in the percentage of children who have a visual acuity level of 20/40 or worse is demonstrated, emphasizing that this increase in visual acuity failure is related to increased myopia rates. The other diagnostic conditions—hyperopia, astigmatism, anisometropia, ocular misalignment, and organic defects—have a fairly constant failure rate that is seemingly independent of age. Between the ages of 16 and 20, most children will have attained their adult refraction, which will remain nearly constant for the next 25 to 30 years.[9-13]

Visual acuity for distant objects improves rapidly from birth until 8 or 9 years with the following approximate progressions: age 1, 20/

---

* As used in this report, the term "corrected" vision denotes an individual's visual ability when tested with whatever lenses, if any, he normally wears.

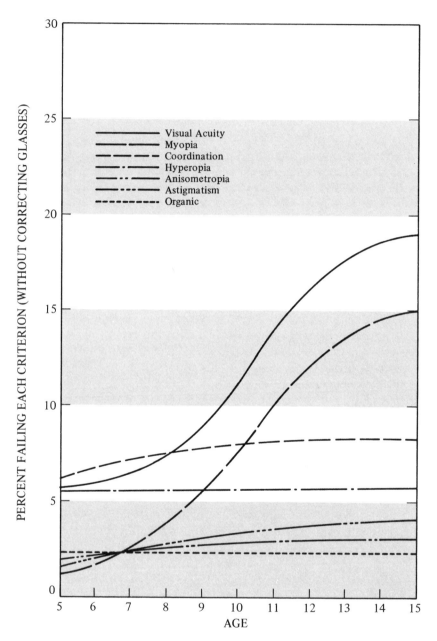

FIGURE 1   Basic changes in visual disorders as related to age. From Blum *et al.*[12] Originally published by the University of California Press; reprinted by permission of the Regents of the University of California.

TABLE 1   Uncorrected Binocular Distance Acuity of Children Age 6-11

Age (years)	Percentage with 20/15 or Better	Percentage with 20/20 or Better	Percentage with 20/70 or Worse
6	22.7	72.7	1.4
7	13.6	.71.6	3.8
8	16.8	75.9	4.2
9	23.0	78.1	5.0
10	28.0	77.8	9.0
11	30.1	73.1	11.5

Source: Adapted from National Center for Health Statistics.[4]

200; age 2, 20/75; age 3, 20/40; age 4, 20/30; age 5, 20/25; and age 6, 20/20.[14,15] Table 1 gives the percentage of children attaining various acuity levels when uncorrected binocular distance vision was tested in the National Health Examination Survey of 1963–1965. At the lower end of the scale (those testing no better than 20/70), there is a consistent increase in defective vision* with age. At the upper end of the scale (those testing at 20/15 or better), consistently better than normal vision increases from age 7 on.

The changes in distance visual acuity with age are shown in Figure 2. The distribution of uncorrected acuity is markedly skewed, which accounts for the large standard deviation and the impression that some children above age 8 have uncorrected acuity better than 20/15. Data are not available to verify the actual distribution of acuities by age. The uncorrected mean visual acuity appears to improve from 5 to 8 years old, but then rapidly declines. This may be due to the inability of young children to respond properly to the Snellen chart and is not necessarily indicative of increased visual acuity. In comparison to these uncorrected data, the distribution for best corrected acuity has a mean about 20/20, with a standard deviation that decreases with age. These data may reflect the common refracting practice of fitting corrective lenses to reach an acuity of 20/20 and of not testing for acuities better than 20/20.

Although children are usually born farsighted, no consistent trend is found by age for poor near acuity (Table 2). This contrasts with the progressive increase in poor distance acuity with increasing age (see Table 1). Defective distance vision is over four times as common as

* Defective vision is used interchangeably with refractive error. The term defective vision does *not* imply that acuity cannot be corrected by appropriate refraction.

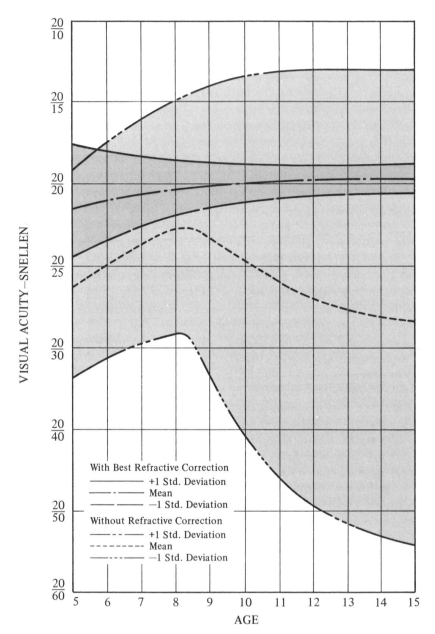

FIGURE 2 Changes in visual acuity (based on the Snellen method) with age. From Blum et al.[12] Originally published by the University of California Press; reprinted by permission of The Regents of the University of California.

TABLE 2   Uncorrected Binocular Near Acuity of Children Age 7–11

Age (years)	Percentage with 14/14 or Better	Percentage with 14/49 or Worse
7	60.8	2.5
8	68.1	2.7
9	74.4	1.9
10	78.3	2.1
11	78.9	3.5

Source: Adapted from National Center for Health Statistics.[4]

defective near vision from age 7 to 11 years. Many screening procedures do not include a test for near visual acuity, because little additional information is gained. Near visual acuity appears to improve
with age.[6,7,16,17]

The percentage of children correctly referred for professional care
varies with the type of screening procedure, the training of the ex-
aminer, the referral criteria, and the age, sex, race, and socioeconomic
status of the children tested. Few published studies segregate data by
age, but a comparison of studies in different age groups indicates an
increase in the percentage of correct referrals with age. Referral rates
for preschoolers (that is, between the ages of 3 and 5) range from
5[18,19] to 21 percent.[20] However, when adjustments are made to com-
pensate for overreferrals (false positive cases), the "correct" referral
rate (true positive cases) for preschoolers is between 5 and 10
percent.[18–25]

Correct referral rates for school-age children range from 16 percent
for first graders up to about 31 percent for children between age 12
and 15.[5,12,17,26,27] Dr. Henry B. Peters[28] concludes that correct
referral rates of approximately 15 percent can be expected for 5-year-
olds, with an increase of 1.6 percent per year for elementary school
children.

The National Health Interview Survey,[13] conducted from July
1965 to June 1966, finds that 15 percent of the 3- to 16-year-old
population and 41.6 percent of the 17- to 24-year-old population
wear corrective lenses. Of the 15 percent wearing corrective lenses in
the younger group, 29.3 percent wear them to improve defective near
vision only, 24.6 percent wear them to improve defective distance
vision only, 39.8 percent wear them for both, and 6.3 percent wear
them for other and unknown reasons. The reliability of these estimates, especially the data on the number who wear lenses to improve

defective near vision, is seriously disputed by experienced clinicians. (It should be noted that these data are based on responses to a household questionnaire and are subject to the inaccuracies inherent in such interview data.)

The only data available on the adequacy of correction is from a study conducted on adults (between age 18 and 79) by the National Health Examination Survey.[29] The survey tested people for distance and near vision, with and without their corrective lenses. Forty-four percent of the entire sample had corrective lenses for defective distance vision. Of this 44 percent, glasses improved acuity for 76 percent, while 19 percent tested the same with and without glasses and 5 percent did better without their glasses. These data suggest, with the exception of those who were being corrected because of esotropia, that their current prescription was no longer appropriate for 24 percent of the national sample examined with correction for distance vision.

Fifty-two percent of the National Health Examination Survey[29] sample had corrective lenses for near vision. Lenses improved acuity for 83 percent of this population. No attempt is made in this study to determine why the remaining 17 percent had decreased acuity. Table 3 shows the proportion of adults reaching or exceeding specific acuity levels for "uncorrected" and "corrected" distance and near vision.

TABLE 3   Uncorrected and Corrected Visual Acuity of Adults

Acuity Levels	Uncorrected (%)	Corrected (%)
Distance		
20/20 or better	53.9	72.9
20/30 or better	69.3	90.6
20/70 or better	83.9	97.7
20/100 or better	93.5	99.2
20/200 or better	97.6	99.6
Near		
14/14 or better	44.7	64.9
14/21 or better	53.6	84.7
14/49 or better	68.2	95.6
14/70 or better	83.9	98.6
14/140 or better	95.7	99.6

Source: Adapted from National Center for Health Statistics.[29]

SEX

Boys generally have better uncorrected distance and near vision than girls[4],[29-33] (Table 4). The differences by sex in the proportion reaching the 20/25 level, or better, are less pronounced in the above studies, but still differ more than would be expected by chance. A study conducted by the National Youth Administration[34] on a population 16 to 24 years old find that the proportion of Negro males scoring at the 20/20 level or better without aid is considerably higher than the proportion of Negro females.

At the poorer end of the scale (20/70 or worse), more girls tend to have defective vision than boys after age 4 (Figure 3). However, when considering severe impairments and blindness (20/200 or worse in the better eye with best correction[1]), school-age boys show a prevalence rate 16 to 26 percent greater than that for girls.[35],[36]

There are similar differences in near visual acuity. The National Health Examination Survey[4] finds that 75 percent of the boys tested had 14/14 or better unaided binocular visual acuity, compared with 69.6 percent of the girls. At the 14/17.5 level or better, differences by sex are much less striking (89.8 percent for boys, compared with 88.5 percent for girls). No consistent patterns by sex emerge in the proportions of boys and girls with near acuity of 14/49 or worse.

Few individual vision screening studies segregate referral data by sex. One study of preschoolers[22] refers 9.7 percent of 172 boys and 10.3 percent of 179 girls, and another study conducted on youths 16 to 21[37] years old refers 17 percent of 116 boys and 34 percent of 153 girls.

Fewer boys wear corrective lenses than girls.[13],[29] The National Health Interview Survey of 1965-1966[13] finds that 13 percent of the

TABLE 4 Percentage of Children with 20/20 or Better Unaided Binocular Vision

Sex	National Health Survey[4] Ages 6-11 (%)	Collins' Study[32] [a] Ages 6-16 (%)
Male	77	65.2
Female	72	60.5

[a]Sample under study was white only. Whites tend to have poorer visual acuity than blacks.
Sources: Adapted from National Center for Health Statistics[4] and Collins.[32]

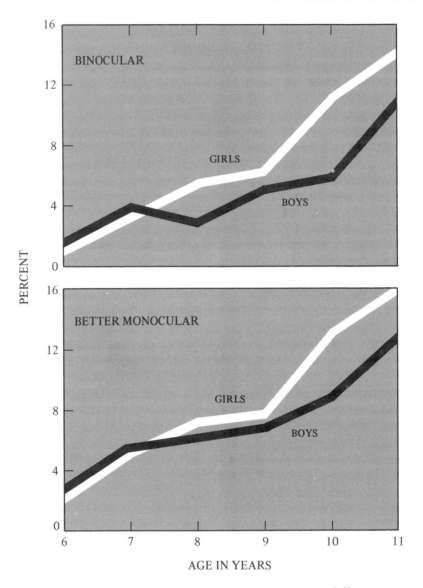

FIGURE 3 Percent of children age 6–11 years, with uncorrected distance visual acuity of 20/70 or worse, by age and sex. From National Center for Health Statistics.[4]

boys between age 3 and 16 wear corrective lenses, compared with 17 percent of the girls in the same age group. As indicated in Figure 4, the percentage of people with corrective lenses increases with age, with the proportion of females exceeding the proportion of males at all age levels. When wearing their usual correction, the differences in vision by sex are essentially eliminated.[29] These data[13,29] do not give good estimates of the need for corrective lenses and leave unanswered the following questions: How many boys and girls should wear glasses but don't? How many children wear glasses that are improperly refracted? How many children wear glasses who really do not need them?

RACE

Blacks of both sexes are found to have better uncorrected visual acuity than whites in all age groups.[30,33,34,38,39] (See Table 5 for a

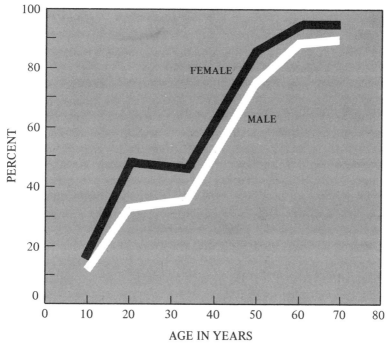

FIGURE 4 Percent of population with corrective lenses, by age and sex. From National Center for Health Statistics.[13]

TABLE 5 Percentage of Children and Young Adults with 20/20 or Better Uncorrected Visual Acuity in at Least One Eye, by Sex and Age[a]

| Race | Farm Security Administration (Low Income)[3] | | | | | | National Youth Administration (Low Income)[34] | | Army Inductees[38] | National Health Survey[30] b | |
	Male (5–9)	Female (5–9)	Male (10–14)	Female (10–14)	Male (15–24)	Female (15–24)	Male (16–24)	Female (16–24)	Male (18–24)	Male (18–24)	Female (18–24)
White	77.1	73.7	78.3	73.2	75.7	69.6	78.7	70.4	78.0	80.3	71.2
Black	86.2	89.3	90.2	92.1	79.6	81.7	80.8	74.8	88.8	75.3	78.8

[a]In years as indicated by range in parentheses under sex.
[b]The percentages for the National Health Survey are given for binocular vision. This survey found that white males scored better than blacks at the 20/20 level or better; however, at the 20/30 level or better, blacks scored significantly better than whites: White—males, 88.8 percent; females, 82.5 percent; Negro—males, 92.7 percent; females, 91.7 percent.
Sources: Adapted from National Center for Health Statistics,[30] Gover and Yankey,[33] National Youth Administration,[34] Karpinos.[38]

summary of available documented findings.) A higher percentage of whites than blacks in all age groups have defective vision of 20/100 or worse (17.2 percent of the white population compared with 8.1 percent of the black population).[30] However, black children have a prevalence rate for severe visual impairment and blindness (20/200 or worse) nearly 20 percent higher than that for white children. The higher rates are chiefly caused by prenatal disorders and/or infectious diseases.[35,36]

At the 14/14 level or better, the National Health Examination Survey of 1960–1962[30] finds no consistent pattern by race and age in the proportion of white and black adults tested without correction; blacks, however, tend to do slightly better. The same also is true at the 14/21 level or better. At the poorer end, a higher proportion of whites (32.7 percent) than blacks (26.5 percent) have acuities of 14/70 or worse; for those between the ages of 18 and 34, however, the differences are not as pronounced. The other studies do not include tests for near vision.

Of the 413 blacks in grades one through eight tested in the Reber study,[5] 13.6 percent are referred for professional care, compared with 19.4 percent of the 2,165 white children tested. Somewhat contradictory data is found by Crane *et al.*[40] Blacks and whites from the first through sixth grades, placed in low- and middle-economic categories based on average monthly rental paid for dwellings, were compared within and between economic strata. From this study findings indicate that a higher proportion of Negro children are referred for professional care than are Caucasian children, regardless of economic status. The children tested by both the National Youth Administration[34] and the Farm Security Administration[33] are in comparable low-income brackets. Both surveys find that without corrective lenses, Negroes score higher on visual acuity tests than Caucasians in all age groups.

The National Health Interview Survey of 1965–1966[13] finds that 16 percent of the white population and 9.2 percent of the nonwhite population between the ages of 3 and 16 have corrective lenses. Nonwhites tend to obtain their corrective lenses later in life than whites; this is particularly true among younger people. Seventy-three percent of the white population, compared with 56.9 percent of the nonwhite population, who wear corrective lenses, obtain them between the ages of 17 and 24. A higher proportion of the white population with corrective lenses tend to wear them all of the time (70.2 percent), compared with 60 percent of the nonwhite population. These findings may be influenced by several factors: (a) better vision and, therefore, less need for visual correction among nonwhite people;[30] (b) lower rates of ophthalmologic care among nonwhite persons;[41,42] and (c) prescription of unnecessary glasses to the white population.

Although Negroes have better uncorrected visual acuity, both distance and near, than whites, their visual acuity with usual correction is substantially poorer, at all age levels, than that of whites. Illustrative findings of the National Health Examination Survey of 1960–1962[29,30] are summarized in Table 6.

SOCIOECONOMIC STATUS

There is little available data relating uncorrected and corrected visual acuity of children to the socioeconomic status of the family. A comparison of individual studies on children between age 5 and 22 from low-income families indicates that between 73 and 79 percent have uncorrected distance visual acuity of 20/20 or better.[33,34,37] Approximately the same proportion of children are found to have unaided vision of 20/20 or better in studies that did not specify the economic background of the children tested.

Schiffer and Hunt[3] find an inverse relationship between severe visual defects in children and size of family income. Three percent of the population sample under age 17 in the less than $2,000 family income group report that they have severe visual defects and blindness compared with 1.3 percent of the children from income groups of $7,000 and over.

The National Health Examination Survey of 1960–1962[30] reveals

TABLE 6   Uncorrected and Corrected Visual Acuity for White and Black Adults

Acuity Level	Uncorrected (%)		Corrected (%)	
	White	Black	White	Black
Distance				
20/20 or better	53.7	56.1	74.2	62.3
20/30 or better	68.4	77.5	91.0	85.0
20/100 or worse	17.2	8.1	2.2	3.4
Near				
14/14 or better	44.4	46.6	66.2	53.0
14/21 or better	52.9	57.8	86.1	72.6
14/70 or worse	32.7	26.5	3.6	11.4

Source: Adapted from National Center for Health Statistics.[29,30]

an inverse relationship between uncorrected visual acuity and combined family income in a national adult sample, age 18 to 79. The proportion of people testing at the 20/20 and 14/14 level or better increases steadily with income size; this rate slows or reverses slightly, however, for those earning $10,000 or more. Rates at the poorer end of the scale (20/100 and 14/70), decrease as family income increases. These trends are strongly related to age, since the lower-income brackets contain a disproportionate number of older people. However, when adjustments are made for age, a direct relationship remains.

Similar data relating income to acuity on a race-specific basis are not available. Although blacks do generally have lower incomes than whites, they also have better mean uncorrected visual acuity as previously described. This appears to contradict the relationship between income and visual acuity. However, this apparent contradiction may be explained by the fact that, at all ages, Negroes have higher prevalence rates for severe visual impairment and blindness.[35,36]

The National Society for the Prevention of Blindness, as cited in Hatfield,[19] finds a rise in referral rates from 4.4 to 5.3 percent for 3- to 6-year-old children. This increase is revealed when the Society compares a vision screening study it conducted in 1963–1964 on a middle-class population of children with a study conducted in 1965–1966 on a group of preschoolers, which included a number of Head Start children. It is concluded that the increase in referral rates may reflect a lower level of health care among the poorer children of the second study, or the differences may merely reflect improved methods of reporting and are not clearly related to socioeconomic factors.. A screening program involving nearly two million Head Start children refers 5–10 percent of the preschoolers examined.[43] This rate is similar to those found in other preschool screening studies and, therefore, offers no evidence that referral rates are higher among the poor.

Crane *et al.*[40] place 1,215 first and sixth graders into five economic categories based on average monthly rental of family homes. They find no evidence of any consistent variation according to economic status in the proportion of children referred for professional eye care.

Although vision studies have been conducted on specified samples of children from low-income families, little research has been conducted that identifies the sample as being from middle- or upper-income families. One study done with high school students reports that the sample was from a white, middle-class, eastern suburb.[44]

Compton[37] compares that project to one conducted on youths (age 16–22) of mixed racial background, from families where the maximum income was $3,130 for four people. Tested without their usual correction, a higher percentage of middle-class youths have defective distance vision than lower-class youths (43 and 27 percent, respectively). However, when tested with their usual correction, only 9 percent of the middle-class youths, compared with 19 percent of the lower-class youths, have visual acuity worse than 20/30.

There is a direct correlation between family income and number of children who have corrective lenses and between income and the adequacy of correction. The National Health Interview Survey of 1965–1966[13] finds that 16.7 percent of the children from families earning $5,000 or more have corrective lenses compared with 11.1 percent of the children from families earning less than $5,000. A study of 16- to 21-year-olds from low-income families[37] reveals that only 56 percent of the youths who needed glasses actually have them. Further, only 60 percent of the youths who have glasses reach acuity levels of 20/30 or better when tested wearing them.

A study conducted with middle-income high school youths[44] reveals that 96 percent of those that needed glasses have them. When wearing their glasses, 83 percent of these youths attain acuity levels of 20/30 or better. Another study,[45] which compared 17- to 18-year-olds from middle- and low-income families, finds that with their usual correction, those youths from middle-class families have significantly better distance acuity than the youths from low-income families. This study makes no attempt to test the youths without their usual correction.

The National Health Examination Survey of 1960–1962,[30] conducted on adults, also finds a direct relationship between size of family income and those who attain higher acuity levels with their usual correction. Table 7 shows that approximately twice as many people who have combined family incomes of $10,000 or more attain acuity levels of 20/20 and 14/14 or better with their usual correction than those with combined family incomes of less than $2,000. Further, there is a 1200 percent difference in the rates for those who have "corrected" vision of no better than 20/100 and 14/70 when families with incomes under $2,000 are compared with those with incomes of $10,000 or more. These data do not include children under age 13.

This same study of adults[30] finds a similar, but even stronger, relationship between social class, as indicated by educational level attained, and acuity levels with usual correction (Table 8).

TABLE 7 "Corrected" Visual Acuity Rates for Adults by Family Income

Combined Family Income	Corrected Distance Vision of 20/20 or Better (%)	Corrected Distance Vision of 20/100 or Worse (%)	Corrected Near Vision of 14/14 or Better (%)	Corrected Near Vision of 14/70 or Worse (%)
Under $2,000	48.0	6.2	40.6	12.3
$2,000–3,999	69.7	2.8	59.4	5.5
$4,000–6,999	79.4	1.5	72.7	2.4
$7,000–9,999	83.1	0.9	75.5	1.3
$10,000 and over	81.6	0.5	73.9	1.2

Source: Adapted from National Center for Health Statistics.[30]

The proportion of the population utilizing the services of ophthalmologists and optometrists[13,42] is directly related to higher educational levels and to higher income levels (Table 9).

GEOGRAPHIC DISTRIBUTION

There is no pattern by geographic location in the distribution of uncorrected acuity levels as defined by the National Health Examination Survey of 1960–1962.[30] When tested with their usual correction, however, adults in the South are found to have poorer vision than those in the West or Northeast (Table 10).

White adults have better corrected vision than blacks in each region; these differences are most pronounced in the South (Figure 5). Regional differences are evident for corrected vision in the black population, but are essentially eliminated when considering corrected vision in the white population.

TABLE 8 "Corrected" Visual Acuity Rates for Adults by Educational Level Attained

Years of Education	Corrected Distance Vision of 20/20 or Better (%)	Corrected Distance Vision of 20/100 or Worse (%)	Corrected Near Vision of 14/14 or Better (%)	Corrected Near Vision of 14/70 or Worse (%)
Under 5	31.2	12.0	20.4	23.5
5–8	57.6	3.1	45.4	6.8
9–12	81.9	1.1	75.5	1.9
13 and over	85.7	0.8	80.4	1.2

Source: Adapted from National Center for Health Statistics.[30]

TABLE 9 Proportion of People Utilizing Professional Eye Care Service by Educational Level and Income

Population as Defined by	Using Ophthalmologist (%)	Using Optometrist (%)	Using Other (%)
Family Income			
Under $5,000	25.2	60.4	12.4
$5,000 and over	35.7	53.7	7.9
Educational Level of Family Head			
12 years or less	27.7	60.2	10.6
13 years or more	47.6	41.5	5.7

Source: Adapted from National Center for Health Statistics.[13,42]

The prevalence of severe impairments and blindness is greater in the South than in the other regions of the United States.[1,46-49] Figure 6, in which the states are ranked in order of their rates of legal blindness, shows these regional variations.

The National Health Interview Survey of 1965-1966[13] finds that a smaller proportion of children living in the South have corrective lenses than children in other regions (Table 11).

In this same study,[13] more rural than urban residents are found to have uncorrected visual acuities of 20/20 and 14/14 or better, and slightly more urban than rural residents are found with uncorrected defective vision of 20/100 and 14/70 or worse (Table 12).

The Farm Security Administration finds that farm families have better uncorrected visual acuity than urban groups, especially between the ages of 20 and 45 years.[33] However, the Children's Bureau study, conducted by Schiffer and Hunt,[3] reports that rural farm children under age 17 show a greater prevalence of uncorrected severe visual

TABLE 10 Percentage of Adults Reaching Specified Corrected Acuity Levels by Three Geographic Regions

Region	Corrected 20/20 or Better (%)	Corrected 20/100 or Worse (%)	Corrected 14/14 or Better (%)	Corrected 14/70 or Worse (%)
Northeast	73.1	2.6	65.5	4.1
West	74.4	1.6	66.5	4.0
South	70.6	2.8	62.1	5.4

Source: Adapted from National Center for Health Statistics.[30]

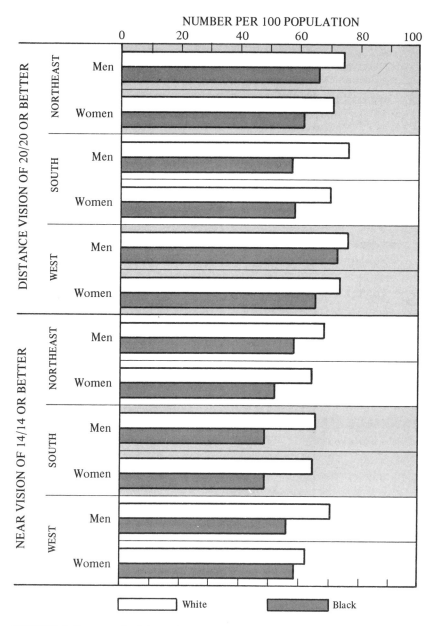

FIGURE 5 Percent of adults with corrected distance and near visual acuity by region for white and black men and women. From National Center for Health Statistics.[30]

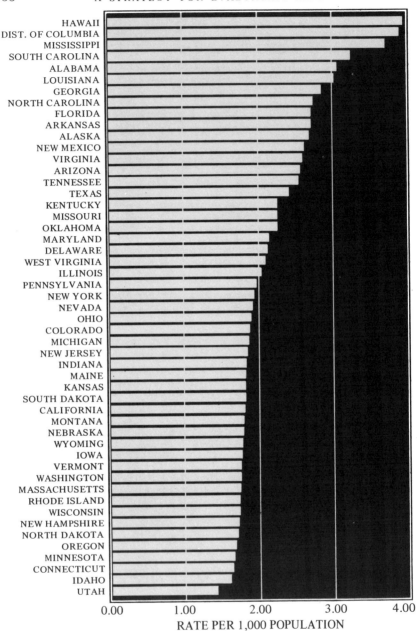

FIGURE 6 States ranked by estimated prevalence rates for legal blindness (1960). From the National Society for the Prevention of Blindness.[1]

TABLE 11 Percentage of People with and without Corrective Lenses by Geographic Region

Region and Age (years)	No Corrective Lenses (%)	Corrective Lenses (%)
Northeast		
All ages, 3 and over	47.4	52.5
3–16	82.6	17.3
North Central		
All ages, 3 and over	49.3	50.6
3–16	81.7	18.1
South		
All ages, 3 and over	57.2	42.8
3–16	88.5	11.3
West		
All ages, 3 and over	52.8	47.0
3–16	85.5	13.9

Source: Adapted from National Center for Health Statistics.[13]

impairment and blindness (2.5 percent) than do children in urban (1.8 percent) and rural nonfarm areas (1.6 percent).

With usual correction, no consistent pattern of urban–rural difference in distance and near visual acuity levels has been noted.[30] In addition, little difference[13] exists between the proportion of children with corrective lenses residing in urban areas (15.4 percent) and those in rural areas (14.3 percent).

TABLE 12 Distribution of Uncorrected Visual Acuities for People Aged 18–79 Years by Area of Residence

Acuity Level	Urban (%)	Rural (%)
Distance		
20/20 or better	52.5	57.1
20/100 or less	16.6	15.0
Near		
14/14 or better	44.1	46.1
14/70 or less	32.0	31.3

Source: Adapted from National Center for Health Statistics.[30]

FUNCTIONAL IMPACT

The relationship between the eye and learning disabilities in children is a very complex subject. Dyslexia, "a child's inability to read with understanding as a result of defects in processing visual symbols,"[50] can play a major role in learning and is a significant social problem. For the purposes of this health services evaluation program, however, we are principally concerned with the relationship between learning and the peripheral eye defects, e.g., refractive errors and muscle imbalance. It is beyond the frame of reference of this discussion to consider the multifactorial psychologic and neurologic variables that are involved in the processing of visual symbols.

The National Society for the Prevention of Blindness estimates[1] prevalence rates for partially seeing school children (visual acuity better than 20/200, but worse than 20/70 in the better eye after correction) as approximately 1 in 500. Children with such visual problems are relatively easy to discover. Those with less obvious refractory errors, however, are more difficult to detect. Rough estimates indicate that 20–25 percent of the 50.7 million children enrolled in public and private schools in the United States have eye disorders that require professional care,[1-4] i.e., are in need of active treatment, glasses, or should be under observation by an eye specialist.

In the past there have been conflicting studies and statements regarding the role of these peripheral eye disorders in reading and learning disorders. Some authors emphasize their importance,[51,52] while others maintain that although peripheral disorders may be contributing factors, they are not critical variables in learning disabilities of children.[53-55] Recently a joint organizational statement on the eye and learning disabilities has been issued[50] by an *ad hoc* committee of the American Academy of Pediatrics, the American Academy of Ophthalmology and Otolaryngology, and the American Association of Ophthalmology with the assistance of the president and past president of the Division for Children with Learning Disabilities. The conclusions reached by the committee are presented in their entirety below:

1. Learning disability and dyslexia, as well as other forms of school underachievement, require a multidisciplinary approach from medicine, education, and psychology in diagnosis and treatment. Eye care should never be instituted in isolation when a patient has a reading problem. Children with learning disabilities have the same incidence of ocular abnormalities, e.g., refractive errors and muscle imbalance,

as children who are normal achievers and reading at grade level.[56-58] These abnormalities should be corrected.

2. Since clues in word recognition are transmitted through the eyes to the brain, it has become common practice to attribute reading difficulties to subtle ocular abnormalities presumed to cause faulty visual perception. Studies have shown that there is no peripheral eye defect that produces dyslexia and associated learning disabilities.[59-60] Eye defects do not cause reversals of letters, words, or numbers.

3. No known scientific evidence supports claims for improving the academic abilities of learning-disabled or dyslexic children with treatment based solely on:

a. visual training (muscle exercises, ocular pursuit, glasses),[61-66]

b. neurologic organizational training (laterality training, balance board, perceptual training).[56-68]

4. Excluding correctable ocular defects, glasses have no value in the specific treatment of dyslexia or other learning problems. In fact, unnecessarily prescribed glasses may create a false sense of security that may delay needed treatment.

5. The teaching of learning-disabled and dyslexic children is a problem of educational science. No one approach is applicable to all children. A change in any variable may result in increased motivation of the child and reduced frustration. Parents should be made aware that mental level and psychological implications are contributing factors to a child's success or failure. Ophthalmologists and other medical specialists should offer their knowledge. This may consist of the identification of specific defects, or simply early recognition.

In summary, the available data indicate that children with learning disabilities have the same incidence of peripheral eye disorders as normal achievers and that such disorders do not directly lead to learning disability. It should be recognized, however, that refractive errors and problems of muscle imbalance should be screened for and corrected at the youngest possible age to ensure clear and efficient visual acuity.

REFERENCES

1. The National Society for the Prevention of Blindness, Inc.: Estimated Statistics on Blindness and Vision Problems. New York, 1966 (1968 supplement included)

2. United States Department of Health, Education, and Welfare: Maternal and Child Health Care Programs (1966). Washington, DC, Government Printing Office, 1966

3. Schiffer CG, Hunt EP: Illness among Children. Children's Bureau, Welfare Administration, Department of Health, Education, and Welfare. Washington, DC, Government Printing Office, 1963

4. National Center for Health Statistics: Visual Acuity of Children, United States. Department of Health, Education, and Welfare. Washington, DC, Government Printing Office, 1970 (PHS Publication No 1000, Series 11, No 101)

5. Reber NJ: Visual screening programs for schools. J Am Optom Assoc 35: 675–680, 1964

6. Borish IM: Clinical Refraction. Second edition. Chicago, The Professional Press, Inc., 1954

7. Cowan A: Normal Eye. Refraction of the eye, The Eye and Its Diseases. Edited by C Berens. Philadelphia, WB Saunders Co, 1949

8. Mann I: Development of the human eye, The Eye and Its Diseases. Edited by C Berens. Philadelphia, WB Saunders Co, 1949

9. Hirsch MJ: The refraction of children, Vision of Children. Edited by MJ Birsch, RE Wick. Philadelphia, Chilton Co, 1963

10. Slataper FJ: Age norms of refraction and vision. Arch Ophthalmol 53:466 479, 1950

11. Brown EVL: Net average yearly changes in refraction of atropinized eyes from birth to beyond middle life. Arch Ophthalmol 19: 719–734, 1938

12. Blum HL, Peters HB, Bettman JW: The Orinda Study. Berkeley, The University of California Press, 1968

13. National Center for Health Statistics: Characteristics of Persons with Corrective Lenses, United States, July 1965–June 1966. Department of Health, Education, and Welfare. Washington, DC, Government Printing Office, 1969 (PHS Publication No 1000, Series 10, No 53)

14. Smith JL: Routine eye examinations of children, Pediatric Ophthalmology. Edited by LB Holt. Philadelphia, Lea & Febiger, 1964

15. Weymouth FW: Visual acuity of children, Vision of Children. Edited by MJ Hirsch, RE Wick. Philadelphia, Chilton Co, 1963

16. Hurst WA: The determination of the near point working distance of the public school child. J Am Optom Assoc 35:610–618, 1964

17. Kempf GA, Collins SD: A special study of the vision of school children. Public Health Rep 43:1713–1739, 1928

18. Colasuonno TM: Preschool vision screening study. Sight-Sav Rev 28:156–162, 1958

19. Hatfield EM: Progress in preschool vision screening. Sight-Sav Rev 37: 194–201, 1967

20. Russell EL, Kada JM, Hufhines DM: Orange County vision screening project. Part II–Ophthalmological evaluation. Sight-Sav Rev 31:215–219, 1961

21. Taubenhaus LJ, Jackson AA: Final Report, Vision Screening of Three through Five Year Old Children, A Research Study. Brookline, Massachusetts Health Department, 1967

22. Hartman E: Preschool health screening in well child clinics. J Sch Health 32:283–291, 1962

23. Kripke SS, Dunbar CA, Zimmerman V: Vision screening of preschool children in mobile clinics in Iowa. Public Health Rep 85:41–44, 1970

24. Moran CT: Preschool vision screening in Louisville. Sight-Sav Rev 28:92–95, 1958

25. Austin C: Mass preschool vision screening. Children 6:58–62, 1959

26. Crane MM, Scobee RG, Foote FM, et al: Study of procedures used for screening elementary school children for visual defects. Am J Public Health 42:1430–1439, 1952

27. Rosen CL: A modified clinic technique in a visual survey of a first grade population. J Sch Health 36:448–449, 1966

28. Peters HB: Vision screening, Vision of Children. Edited by MJ Hirsch, RE Wick. Philadelphia, Chilton Co, 1963

29. National Center for Health Statistics: Binocular Visual Acuity of Adults, United States, 1960–1962. Department of Health, Education, and Welfare. Washington, DC, Government Printing Office, 1964 (PHS Publication No 1000, Series 11, No 3

30. National Center for Health Statistics: Binocular Visual Acuity of Adults by Region and Selected Demographic Characteristics, United States, 1960–1962. Department of Health, Education, and Welfare. Washington, DC, Government Printing Office, 1967 (PHS Publication No 1000, Series 11, No 25)

31. National Center for Health Statistics: History and Examination Findings Related to Visual Acuity among Adults. Department of Health, Education, and Welfare. Washington, DC, Government Printing Office, 1968 (PHS Publication No 1000, Series 11, No 28)

32. Collins SD: The eyesight of the school child as determined by the Snellen test. Public Health Rep 39:3013–3027, 1924

33. Gover M, Yaukey JB: Physical impairments of members of low-income farm families—11,499 persons in 2,477 Farm Security Administration borrower families, 1940. Public Health Rep 59:1163–1184, 1944

34. National Youth Administration: The Health Status of NYA Youth. Federal Security Agency, Public Health Service. Washington, DC, Government Printing Office, 1942

35. Kerby CE: Causes of blindness in children of school age. Sight-Sav Rev 28:10–21, 1958

36. Hatfield EM: Causes of blindness in school children. Sight-Sav Rev 33:218–233, 1963

37. Compton AS: Health study of adolescents enrolled in the Neighborhood Youth Corps. Public Health Rep 84:585–596, 1969

38. Karpinos BD: Racial differences in visual acuity. Public Health Rep 75:1045–1050, 1960

39. Karpinos BD: Visual acuity of selectees and army inductees. Hum Biol 16:1–14, 1944

40. Crane MM, Foote FM, Scobee RG, et al: Screening School Children for Visual Defects. Department of Health, Education, and Welfare. Washington, DC, Government Printing Office, 1954 (CB Publication 345)

41. National Center for Health Statistics: Volume of Physician Visits, United States, July 1966–June 1967. Department of Health, Education, and Welfare. Washington, DC, Government Printing Office, 1968 (PHS Publication No 1000, Series 10, No 49)

42. National Center for Health Statistics: Characteristics of Patients of Selected
    Types of Medical Specialists and Practitioners, United States, July 1963–
    June 1964. Department of Health, Education, and Welfare. Washington, DC,
    Goverment Printing Office, 1966 (PHS Publication No 1000, Series 10, No
    28)
43. North AF: Vision care in Project Head Start. Sight-Sav Rev 37:153–156,
    1967
44. Rogers KD, Reese G: Health studies–presumably normal high school stu-
    dents. I. Physical appraisal. Am J Dis Child 108:572–600, 1964
45. Farrell E: Relationship between socioeconomic status and visual acuity.
    Nurs Res 18:538–541, 1969
46. National Center for Health Statistics: Characteristics of Visually Impaired
    Persons, United States, July 1963–June 1964. Department of Health, Educa-
    tion, and Welfare. Washington, DC, Government Printing Office, 1968
    (PHS Publication No 1000, Series 10, No 46)
47. National Center for Health Statistics: Prevalence of Selected Impairments,
    United States, July 1963–June 1965. Department of Health, Education, and
    Welfare. Washington, DC, Government Printing Office, 1968 (PHS Publica-
    tion No 1000, Series 10, No 48)
48. Hurlin RG, Perkins WM: Regional differences in the prevalence of blindness.
    Soc Secur Bull 13:9–10, 1950
49. Hurlin RG: Estimated prevalence of blindness in the United States, July
    1952. Soc Secur Bull 16:8–11, 1953
50. Joint Organizational Statement. The eye and learning disabilities. Newsl Am
    Acad Pediatr 23:(Suppl), 1972
51. Robinson HM: Why Pupils Fail in Reading. Chicago, University of Chicago
    Press, 1946
52. Eames TH: Comparison of eye conditions among 1000 reading failures,
    500 ophthalmic patients and 150 unselected children. Am J Ophthalmol
    31:713–717, 1948
53. Flom BC: The Optometrists's role in the reading field, Vision of Children.
    Edited by MJ Hirsch, RE Wick. Philadelphia, Chilton Co, 1963
54. Nicholls JVV: Reading difficulties in children, Refraction. Edited by BC
    Gettes. Boston, Little, Brown and Company, 1965
55. Jampolsky A, Grown KA: Symposium: Reading disabilities in children.
    Cal Med 83:79–81, 1955
56. Flax N: Visual function in learning disabilities. J Learn Disabilities 1:551–
    556, 1968
57. Bettman JW Jr., Stern EL, Whitsell LJ, et al: Cerebral dominance in develop-
    mental dyslexia: Role of ophthalmologist. Arch Ophthalmol 78:722–729,
    1967
58. Norn MS, Rindziunski E, Skydsgaard H: Ophthalmologic and orthoptic
    examinations of dyslectics. Acta Ophthalmol 47:147–160, 1969
59. Goldberg HK, Drash PW: The disabled reader. J Pediatr Ophthalmol 5:11–24,
    1968
60. Goldberg HK: The ophthalmologist looks at the reading problem. Am J
    Ophthalmol 47(Part I):67–74, 1959
61. Robbins MP: Test of the Doman–Delacato rationale with retarded readers.
    JAMA 202:389–393, 1967

62. Cohen HJ, Birch HG, Taft LT: Some considerations for evaluating the Doman–Delacato "Patterning" method. Pediatrics 45:302–314, 1970

63. Freeman RD: Controversy over "patterning" as a treatment for brain damage in children. JAMA 202:385–388, 1967

64. Committee on the Handicapped Child: Doman–Delacato treatment of neurologically handicapped children. Am Acad Pediatr Newsl 19 (Supplement), 1968

65. Goldberg HK: Role of patching in learning. J. Pediatr Ophthalmol 6:123–124, 1969

66. Goldberg HK, Arnott W: Ocular motility in learning disabilities. J Learn Disabilities 3:160–162, 1970

67. Rosen CL: An experimental study of visual perceptual training and reading achievement in first grade. Percept Mot Skills 22:979–986, 1966

68. Smith HM: Motor acitivity and perceptual development. J Health-Phys-Recreation 39:28–33, 1968

BIBLIOGRAPHY

Armed Forces–NRC Committee on Vision: Proceedings of Spring Meeting 1965: The Measurement of Visual Function. Edited by MA Whitcomb, W Benson. Washington, DC, National Academy of Sciences, National Research Council, 1968

Council on Pediatric Practice: Standards of Child Health Care. Evanston, Illinois, Academy of Pediatrics, Inc, 1967

Goldberg HK, Shiffman G: Fundamentals of Dyslexia. New York, Grune & Stratton, Inc (in press)

Keeney AH, Keeney VT: Dyslexia, Diagnosis and Treatment of Reading Disorders. St Louis, The CV Mosby Co, 1968

Myklebust H: Progress in Learning Disabilities, Vol. I. New York, Grune & Stratton, Inc, 1968

Mykelbust H: Progress in Learning Disabilities, Vol. II. New York, Grune & Stratton, Inc (in press)

National Society for the Prevention of Blindness: Vision Screening of Children. A Statement of Principles Established by the National Society for the Prevention of Blindness, Inc, New York, 1969

FOUR

Iron-Deficiency Anemia

SUMMARY

Because proper diet or supplemental iron can prevent iron deficiency, anemia is an excellent tracer in both preschool-age children and females of child-bearing age. The condition is useful also as an indicator of how well a system screens for particular conditions and challenges the providers of health care in the appropriate use of laboratory procedures. The responsible medical providers must not only prescribe and rigorously follow up treatment but, with proper dietary and health counseling, can prevent recurrences of iron-deficiency anemia in which blood loss is not the cause. Where blood loss is the primary cause, the use of inpatient facilities and general diagnostic skills can be assessed.

CLASSIFICATION

Although the exact prevalence of iron-deficiency anemia in the general United States population is unknown, the prevalence of anemia, unspecified as to etiology, is estimated to be between 5 and 10 percent. This range is due to the variability in criteria used for anemia, a factor that affects all of the data presented herein. It is generally agreed that iron deficiency is the most prevalent nutritional deficiency in this country and the most common cause of anemia. However, only by employing specific tests for iron deficiency can anemia be accurately classified.

EPIDEMIOLOGY

Age and Sex Before puberty there is little difference in the prevalence of anemia by sex. However, age appears to be a very important factor, with the highest rates found in infants 6–24 months of age. By age 3 the prevalence of a hemoglobin concentration of 10 g/100 ml or less is reduced by a factor of 0.5 to approximately 10 percent. With increasing age there is a progressive decline in prevalence to 2 percent in 5- to 13-year-olds. Following puberty the distribution of anemia is both age- and sex-related, with adolescent and adult females showing higher prevalence rates than males. This sex differential decreases in older adults, as there is a progressive decrease in the mean hematocrit of adult males with increasing age. The converse, however, is true for females.

Race In general, the highest prevalence of anemia is found in the nonwhite population. These differences are most striking for black infants, 4 months through 1 year of age, who have mean hemoglobin values 0.5–1 g/100 ml lower than whites. These racial differences are noted in national data for all age and sex groups, except males age 18–24. The prevalence of anemia in the white population is generally one half that found in blacks of the same sex and age.

Socioeconomic Status Despite the paucity of reliable data relating anemia to socioeconomic status, the trend indicates an inverse relationship between the prevalence of anemia and social class. National Health Survey data document higher mean hematocrits with increasing family income for the black but not the white population, while the National Nutritional Survey, using a composite poverty index and hemoglobin concentration, shows this same relationship for the total population sampled. Case studies of private and service patients generally reinforce these relationships and emphasize the very low rates of anemia in selected private patient populations.

Other Variables Pregnant women not receiving iron supplements show very high rates of anemia. In large maternity populations, 20–50 percent are found to have a hemoglobin value of 11 g/100 ml or less.

Furthermore, there is an inverse relationship between birthweight and the prevalence of anemia in infants that extends throughout the first 2 years of life. Parity, birth order, and spacing of pregnancies are additional pregnancy-related factors that are important determinants in the development of anemia in the mother and infant.

Functional Impact   Iron-deficiency anemia is merely a symptom of a more general nutritional and environmental problem. Although it is often difficult, particularly in adults, to be certain that the symptoms usually attributed to anemia—easy fatigability and general asthenia—are indeed due to a mild iron deficiency, recent work with children suggests significant systemic effects from mild to moderate iron deficiency: Preliminary studies on iron-deficient children and controls have exhibited significant differences in attentiveness and learning ability. When iron deficiency was corrected, learning patterns and attentiveness improved. Further, animal studies suggest that iron deficiency results in enzymatic cellular defects. In addition to these more subtle findings, it is well known that severe chronic iron deficiency anemia has significant adverse effects on the circulatory system that are relatively uncommon in mild iron-deficiency anemia.

A MINIMAL-CARE PLAN FOR ANEMIA IN CHILDREN (TO AGE 5)

I. Screening

   A. *Method*.   Hemoglobin, standard hematocrit, or microhematocrit.
   B. *Criteria.*   Up to age 5 years, fail if hematocrit is 33 percent or less, hemoglobin 11 g/100 ml or less, or mean corpuscular hemoglobin concentration (MCHC), $\frac{Hb}{Hct}$, is less than 33 percent.
   C. *Time and frequency.*   Once during 6 to 12 months of age and annually thereafter.

II. Evaluation

   A. *History.*   (1) Family history of anemia; (2) birthweight; (3) general diet and milk intake, specifying cow's milk or formula.
   B. *Physical examination.*   (1) Height and weight; (2) pulse rate;

(3) jaundice; (4) cardiac: standard description; (5) abdominal: standard description.

C. *Laboratory.* (1) Any of the following: repeat hemoglobin or hematocrit; red blood count (RBC) indices; red blood cell morphology; serum iron, total iron-binding capacity, and percent transferrin saturation; (2) stool examination for occult blood.

III. Diagnosis

A. *Iron-deficiency anemia, definite.* Based upon low serum iron and increased iron-binding capacity with a transferrin saturation of less than 15 percent.

B. *Iron-deficiency anemia, presumptive.* Based on morphology or RBC indices showing hypochromic microcytic red cells.

C. *Anemia, type unspecified.*

IV. Management

A. *Definite and presumptive iron-deficiency anemia.* (1) Iron: ferrous sulfate, gluconate, or fumarate to provide 2 mg/kg of elemental iron by mouth three times a day; (2) dietary program: limit milk to 1 pint/day with adequate total caloric intake; (3) treatment of intestinal parasites and gastrointestinal blood loss.

B. *Anemia, type unspecified.* Further evaluation including (1) complete blood count (CBC); (2) reticulocyte count; (3) platelet count; (4) bilirubin; (5) Coombs; (6) Hb electrophoresis; (7) serum iron and iron-binding capacity; (8) blood lead level; (9) repeat stools for occult blood loss and gastrointestinal evaluation as indicated.

C. *Follow-up for definite or presumptive iron-deficiency anemia.* (1) Repeat hemoglobin or hematocrit 3–4 weeks after initiating iron therapy; (2) continue iron therapy 4–6 weeks after hemoglobin or hematocrit is normal.

D. *Outcome criteria.* Hemoglobin greater than 11 g/100 ml and hematocrit greater than 33 percent.

PATHOGENESIS

Iron-deficiency is considered the most widespread nutritional deficiency in the United States[1-4] and the most common cause of anemia. Although the general prevalence of this specific anemia is unknown, the prevalence of unspecified anemias, as measured by hemoglobin and hematocrit values, is estimated to be between 5 and 10 percent.

Almost 75 percent of the total body iron of the newborn child is found in hemoglobin. The remaining iron is distributed in myoglobin, enzymes, and as storage iron in the liver and spleen. The premature infant has greater iron needs than the term infant because of lower total iron content at birth and a proportionately greater postnatal growth rate. By no later than 3 months of age, full-term infants require a source of exogenous dietary iron.* Based on an absorption rate of 10 percent of dietary iron, the daily infant requirement is calculated at approximately 1 mg iron per kilogram of body weight in order to prevent deficiency.[5-6] The Committee on Nutrition of the American Academy of Pediatrics has recently recommended that all infants receive an iron supplemented formula[7] to meet these needs during the first year of life.

The average adult diet contains 10–15 mg iron, 0.5–1.5 mg of which is absorbed daily. Women have increased needs of daily iron intake[8]: The menstruating woman must absorb 0.7–2.0 mg to maintain balance, and the pregnant woman requires an even greater daily intake because of iron transferred to the fetus and placental structure, additional requirements to meet the expansion of blood plasma volume, and blood loss at parturition. In the last two trimesters of pregnancy iron requirements are approximately 3–7.5 mg/day. Similarly, postpartum iron requirements remain high in the lactating woman.

The early manifestations of iron-deficiency anemia are decreased hemoglobin concentration, normal or slightly depressed plasma iron levels, normal or slightly increased iron-binding capacity, and a decrease in the percentage of transferrin saturated. With prolonged iron deficiency, hemoglobin concentration decreases further, plasma iron is almost invariably low, and iron-binding capacity is high. The erythrocytes, initially normocytic and normochromic, gradually become microcytic and hypochromic as anemia develops. This sequence may be modified by the rate of iron depletion; rapid depletion is often coupled with normocytic anemia.

Diet is an important factor in the development of iron deficiency in infants. In the past, correlations between heavy milk consumption and the development of anemia in infants were attributed entirely to the low iron content of milk. Recent studies, however, have indicated that consumption of large quantities of homogenized cow's milk leads

*N. J. Smith, personal communication, March 28, 1972.

to occult blood loss.[9] The cause of this phenomenon remains unexplained.

In adults, diet is rarely the only cause for iron-deficiency anemia. Food idiosyncracies or pica (especially clay and starch ingestion by pregnant women) are contributing factors in population groups with enhanced iron requirements. Also, many women fail to provide in their diet the extra iron needed to replace that lost through menstruation. This combination of inadequate diet and blood loss in women of childbearing age is one of the most common causes of iron-deficiency anemia. In adult males, however, iron-deficiency anemia, with rare exception, is an indication of pathologic blood loss.

METHODOLOGICAL CONSIDERATIONS

Estimates of iron-deficiency anemia prevalence depend on the hematologic tests and criteria used to screen for anemia. Prevalence figures derived from the literature vary, however, because of a lack of standardized techniques for diagnosis and an absence of uniform criteria for interpretation of the tests.

Hematocrit and hemoglobin determinations are the simplest and most reliable screening procedures. A simple microhematocrit determination proves to be both accurate and reliable when compared with the standard Wintrobe method.[10-12] Many large-scale surveys, especially in pediatric populations, use only these screening measures, which necessitates estimating the proportion of anemias that are due to iron deficiency. Specific tests for iron deficiency, such as plasma or serum iron determinations and measurement of iron-binding capacity and percent saturation of transferrin, provide the only reliable tools for determining the true prevalence of iron-deficiency anemia.

It is difficult to establish a standard hemoglobin concentration or hematocrit level below which anemia can be said to exist. Because the range of "normal" hematologic values is wide, what is optimal for one age-specific group might be considered deficient for another. Again, interpretation of data from different studies is difficult because of the lack of uniformity in criteria and failure to describe adequately the population at risk, although the impact of age and sex on hemoglobin and hematocrit levels is usually accounted for in the setting of standards. The use of different laboratory techniques for hemoglobin and hematocrit determination is yet another source of interstudy variation.

EPIDEMIOLOGY

AGE AND SEX

Many investigators have reported the distribution of anemia by age and sex, and because the effects of sex on the distribution of anemia vary with the age group studied, these two variables are generally combined. Information on age and sex in infants and children is clear and well documented. The influence of these factors on the distribution of anemia in adult and geriatric populations is less clear, largely due to inconsistent criteria.

Sex does not appear to be a significant factor before the onset of puberty, with equal rates of anemia reported for both males and females of the same age.[13-16] Age, however, is an extremely important factor. Table 1 summarizes data collected from 36 comprehensive health projects for children and youth in 1968.[17] The population at highest risk is the group age 6-24 months, a finding not inconsistent with those of other investigators.[8, 15, 18-24] By 2-3 years old, the risk diminishes,[5, 8, 21, 22] and from 4 through 14 years, prevalence rates are substantially reduced.[8, 16, 22-26] These age trends may be the result of using a uniform criterion of hemoglobin (10 g/100 ml or less) to designate anemia. If more realistic criteria are applied (11 g/100 ml for the first two years of life, 12 g/100 ml to age 6, and 12-13 g/100 ml for adolescents), little decrease in the incidence of iron-deficiency anemia is observed in high risk populations.*

Following puberty, distributions of hemoglobin and hematocrit values appear to be affected by sex as well as by age. Studies of adolescents and young adults report lower hemoglobin and hematocrit levels in women than in men.[16, 27-35]

In a study on the hemoglobin levels of 268 adolescent patients evaluated at the University of Alabama Medical Center, Daniel and Rowland[30] find 3 percent of the boys and 4 percent of the girls tested had hemoglobin values less than 11 g/100 ml and were classified as anemic. Kirschenfeld and Tew,[36] in a family practice in rural Alabama, find anemia rates to be 20.7 percent for women (Hb < 11 g/100 ml) and 13.1 percent for men (Hb < 12 g/100 ml).

Data from the National Health Survey of 1960-1962[28] present a cumulative percentage distribution of hematocrit in adults by age and sex, without setting specific criteria for anemia (Table 2). Using a com-

---

*N. Smith, personal communication, December 1971.

TABLE 1 Percentage of Children in 1968 Children and Youth Survey with Hemoglobin Concentrations 10 g/100 ml or Less

Age (years)	No. of Children	Percent with Hb Concentration (10 g/100 ml or less)
0–0.5	1,722	13.6
0.5–1	1,293	22.1
1–2	1,813	28.5
2–3	1,245	9.2
3–4	1,045	3.2
4–5	1,107	2.4
5–13	4,873	1.9

Source: Maternal and Child Health Service.[17]

monly employed definition of anemia (a hematocrit level below 33 percent in women and below 35 percent in men), however, women show a much higher prevalence of anemia than do men in all age groups under 55.

Studies of geriatric populations indicate a high prevalence of anemia, with a notable increase in risk among males. Differences in anemia rates by sex do not appear as marked among the aged as in younger adults. However, the National Health Survey[28] finds that mean hematocrit levels decrease with increasing age for men over 24 years. Mean hematocrit levels for women 18 and over increased until age 55–64, after which they decline. Although women have a lower mean hematocrit than men in every age group, the difference is much less marked with increasing age (Table 3).

The National Nutrition Survey, released as a preliminary report to Congress in April 1971,[29] provides the most extensive data currently available on the prevalence of anemia. The survey, aimed at determining nutritional levels of low-income families, however, does not provide a cross section of the U.S. population: Hemoglobin levels were determined on 32,669 individuals from a total of 10 states and New York City. The general prevalence of anemia is found to be between 5 and 10 percent, as defined by deficient hemoglobin levels (see Table 4 for standards). Unfortunately, specific tests for iron deficiency are not correlated with the hemoglobin data for this preliminary report.

The survey reports on hemoglobin deficiencies by both specific age (Table 5) and sex groups (Table 6), but not by age and sex combined.

TABLE 2   Cumulative Percent Hematocrit Distribution, by Age and Sex, in the United States, 1960–1962

Sex and Hematocrit Level	Age Group (years)							
	18–24	25–34	35–44	45–54	55–64	65–74	75–79	Total
Men								
Under 35.0	0.4	0.0	0.9	0.4	0.8	1.0	1.9	0.6
35.0–36.9	1.7	0.3	1.1	0.7	1.8	1.6	7.3	1.3
37.0–38.9	2.4	0.8	1.6	2.9	2.8	4.6	11.3	2.5
39.0–40.9	3.4	2.6	5.6	6.4	6.3	11.2	16.7	5.8
41.0–42.9	12.6	9.1	11.3	14.5	16.2	21.9	22.7	13.6
43.0–44.9	27.0	23.5	27.8	33.6	33.3	34.8	36.3	29.6
45.0–46.9	47.1	46.2	52.6	52.3	56.6	57.0	56.9	51.7
47.0–48.9	72.5	70.2	72.7	72.5	76.6	77.1	83.6	73.4
49.0–50.9	87.3	88.5	88.4	88.2	88.6	89.1	92.8	88.5
51.0–52.9	94.8	95.9	95.2	94.6	94.9	95.9	97.5	95.3
53.0–54.9	98.8	98.7	98.3	98.2	98.7	97.9	99.0	98.5
55.0–56.9	99.8	99.6	99.3	99.4	99.4	98.6	99.0	99.4
57.0 and over	100.0	100.0	100.0	100.0	100.0	100.0	100.0	100.0
Women								
Under 31.0	1.0	0.9	1.1	1.1	–	1.1	2.2	0.9
31.0–32.9	2.2	2.1	2.1	2.0	0.2	1.1	4.5	1.8
33.0–34.9	5.0	4.3	4.1	3.6	0.7	1.9	4.5	3.5
35.0–36.9	11.3	9.0	7.8	6.2	2.0	3.8	6.2	7.0
37.0–38.9	22.5	19.3	16.4	13.7	4.3	10.3	8.6	14.9
39.0–40.9	37.5	36.1	32.7	28.7	17.1	25.1	18.7	30.0
41.0–42.9	62.0	59.7	56.9	52.3	37.5	42.4	33.5	52.6
43.0–44.9	82.5	78.3	75.6	72.0	61.2	64.2	71.7	73.2
45.0–46.9	92.4	90.7	88.6	86.9	84.2	82.4	87.6	87.9
47.0–48.9	97.2	97.5	95.4	94.7	93.3	94.0	93.1	95.4
49.0–50.9	99.5	98.7	99.4	98.9	98.6	96.3	97.5	98.7
51.0–52.9	99.7	99.6	99.8	99.8	99.2	98.8	97.5	99.5
53.0 and over	100.0	100.0	100.0	100.0	100.0	100.0	100.0	100.0

Source: National Center for Health Statistics.[28]

In the adult group (age 17–49) 1.8 percent of the sample are hemoglobin deficient (criteria: for males, under 12 g/100 ml; for females, under 10 g/100 ml). Data shown in Table 6 indicate that, as a group, males have a higher prevalence of hemoglobin deficiency than do females. This finding contradicts previous studies and cannot be explained by available data. However, some hematologists do question the criteria that have been used, particularly those for adult males.[27]

RACE

The prevalence of iron-deficiency anemia in the United States is generally higher among the nonwhite population. Investigators have long

TABLE 3 Mean Hematocrit in Adults, by Sex and Age in the United States, 1960–1962

Age Group (years)	Mean Hematocrit (ml %)	
	Men	Women
18–24	46.7	41.4
25–34	47.0	41.8
35–44	46.6	42.0
45–54	46.5	42.5
55–64	46.1	43.7
65–74	45.8	43.2
75–79	45.1	43.1
TOTAL	46.5	42.4

Source: National Center for Health Statistics.[28]

been aware of racial differences in hemoglobin levels. In 1936 Munday *et al.*[37] found that the average hemoglobin values for white infants were 0.5–1 g/100 ml higher than those for black infants between age 4 months and 1 year. No racial differences are observed in hemoglobin curves until after the third month, suggesting that this pattern was due to differences in dietary iron intake. In 1946 Milam and Muench[38] reported similar differences in values for a sample of 2,168 white and 861 black subjects. They conclude that mean hemoglobin levels for black persons, both under and over 12 years of age, were 0.5–1 g below those of white counterparts.

TABLE 4 Criteria for Hemoglobin Deficient and Low Hemoglobin by Age and Sex for Nutrition Survey in Eight States and New York City, 1968–1970 (Preliminary)

Age Group	Deficient	Low	Acceptable
6–23 months	<9.0	9.0–9.9	⩾10.0
2–5 years	<10.0	10.0–10.9	⩾11.0
6–12 years	<10.0	10.0–11.4	⩾11.5
13–16 years			
male	<12.0	12.0–12.9	⩾13.0
female	<10.0	10.0–11.4	⩾11.5
Over 16 years			
male	<12.0	12.0–13.9	⩾14.0
female	<10.0	10.0–11.9	⩾12.0
Pregnant, third trimester	<9.5	9.5–10.9	⩾11.0

Source: Center for Disease Control.[29]

TABLE 5 Nutrition Surveys Comparing Number, Percent Deficient, and Percent Deficient and Low Hemoglobin, by Age, in Eight States and New York City, 1968–1970 (Preliminary)ᵃ

Age Group (years)

Area	6 and Under			6–9			10–16			17–49			50–59			60 and Over		
	Number	Deficient (%)	Deficient and Low (%)	Number	Deficient (%)	Deficient and Low (%)	Number	Deficient (%)	Deficient and Low (%)	Number	Deficient (%)	Deficient and Low (%)	Number	Deficient (%)	Deficient and Low (%)	Number	Deficient (%)	Deficient and Low (%)
New York State	302	6.6	20.2	339	0.0	6.5	486	1.6	7.2	1,035	0.4	9.8	277	0.7	9.4	366	2.5	13.2
Kentucky	183	9.3	26.2	164	0.0	13.4	239	2.9	13.4	352	2.3	19.6	120	2.5	19.2	197	6.6	22.8
Michigan	115	2.6	10.4	325	0.9	19.4	515	2.9	17.1	582	1.4	19.3	122	0.8	16.4	250	2.8	23.2
New York City	301	6.3	19.9	255	1.2	15.7	388	2.6	13.9	693	1.0	16.9	121	5.0	17.4	124	1.6	21.8
West Virginia	101	1.0	6.9	186	0.5	10.2	254	2.4	9.5	431	1.6	14.6	124	0.8	12.1	200	1.5	18.0
California	565	5.7	14.7	654	0.2	6.5	924	1.4	8.3	1,742	0.9	10.4	346	1.4	13.2	553	1.4	12.2
Washington	122	0.0	2.5	275	0.0	3.6	427	0.5	6.8	804	1.2	11.0	161	0.6	9.3	257	1.2	14.8
South Carolina	562	16.5	35.7	592	5.9	44.2	1,082	6.6	31.0	1,006	6.6	38.4	226	6.6	36.2	280	7.9	42.5
Massachusetts	385	4.4	13.8	498	0.0	6.0	717	1.4	6.3	1,388	1.2	10.4	248	0.4	7.7	298	0.0	9.4
TOTAL	2,636	7.7	20.0	3,288	1.3	15.5	5,032	2.8	14.3	8,033	1.8	15.7	1,745	2.0	15.3	2,525	2.7	18.5

ᵃFor standards used in these surveys, see Table 4.
Source: Center for Disease Control.[29]

TABLE 6 Nutrition Surveys Comparing Number, Percent Deficient, and Percent Deficient and Low Hemoglobin, by Sex, in 10 States and New York City, 1968–1970 (Preliminary)[a]

	Male			Female		
Area	Number	Deficient (%)	Deficient and Low (%)	Number	Deficient (%)	Deficient and Low (%)
Texas	1,371	N.A.[b]	21.2	1,880	N.A.	17.6
Louisiana	1,806	N.A.	42.0	2,539	N.A.	35.7
New York State	1,277	2.3	12.8	1,446	0.9	8.0
Kentucky	568	5.6	23.2	688	2.3	15.6
Michigan	797	2.9	21.6	1,099	1.2	16.4
New York City	780	2.8	17.2	1,086	2.3	16.9
West Virginia	540	2.0	16.9	752	0.9	9.6
California	1,986	2.0	11.7	2,711	1.3	9.2
Washington	900	0.7	10.4	1,097	0.8	7.8
South Carolina	1,550	9.9	42.8	2,183	6.8	33.0
Massachusetts	1,584	1.8	10.7	1,942	0.9	7.8
TOTAL	13,159	3.5	22.0	17,423	2.2	16.9

[a]For standards used in these surveys, see Table 4.
[b]N.A.–Not available
Source: Center for Disease Control.[29]

More recent surveys have specifically identified the black child as being at a high risk for anemia.[22, 37–44] Further, Hutcheson[41] finds that black children of all ages have hematocrits below 31 percent more often than do white children. Forty percent of black, compared to 27 percent of white, 1-year-olds have hematocrits at or under 31 percent, a racial difference that is statistically significant. Analysis of the nutritional status of 642 New York children by Christakis *et al.*[39] reveals no white children with hemoglobin values under 10 g/100 ml or hematocrit under 35 percent. In contrast, 3.1 percent of black children have deficient hemoglobin values (i.e., below 10 g/100 ml) and 15.6 percent have hematocrits under 35 percent.

Several recent studies have also indicated that black adults have higher rates of anemia than do whites. Kirschenfeld and Tew,[36] in a study of 300 consecutive new outpatients in rural Alabama, find that anemia occurred approximately twice as frequently in black as in white patients. Similarly, the 1961–1962 National Health Survey[28] finds significantly greater percentages of black women with low hematocrit levels (Table 7). Moreover, in every age group except 18- to 24-year-old men, whites have a higher mean hematocrit than

TABLE 7 Cumulative Percent Hematocrit Distribution, by Sex and Race in the United States, 1960–1962

Hematocrit Level (%)	Men		Women	
	White	Black	White	Black
Under 29.0	0.1	–	0.4	0.8
29.0–30.9	0.1	–	0.6	3.3
31.0–32.9	0.5	0.5	1.3	5.8
33.0–34.9	0.6	0.5	2.7	9.4
35.0–36.9	1.3	1.6	6.0	15.5
37.0–38.9	2.4	3.8	13.6	25.8
39.0–40.9	5.4	10.3	28.8	42.8
41.0–42.9	13.1	19.6	51.0	65.6
43.0–44.9	28.3	42.0	72.1	84.0
45.0–46.9	51.1	57.0	87.3	94.5
47.0–48.9	73.6	74.5	95.1	97.7
49.0–50.9	88.6	90.4	98.6	99.3
51.0–52.9	95.3	96.2	99.4	99.7
53.0–54.9	98.5	98.7	99.8	99.8
55.0–56.9	99.3	99.8	99.9	99.8
57.0 and over	100.0	99.9	99.9	99.9

Source: National Center for Health Statistics.[28]

do blacks of the same sex. A study by McDonough[45] *et al.* presents similar hematocrit data by age, sex, and race, exhibiting significantly lower hematocrit values for blacks than whites in both sexes. This is constant for every age group except 15- to 34-year-old men.

Information concerning anemia in racial groups other than blacks and whites is sparse and incomplete. Available data does suggest that the prevalence of anemia is higher in Puerto Ricans, Mexican Americans, and American Indians than in whites, but lower than in black populations.[23, 29, 39, 46–52] The National Nutrition Survey data confirm this trend, despite marked variation by racial group between states (Table 8).

SOCIOECONOMIC STATUS

There is a dearth of reliable data relating the distribution of anemia to socioeconomic status. In general, the available literature indicates that the prevalence of anemia is inversely related to social class.[20, 23, 29, 40, 53–58]

The 1960–1962 National Health Survey[28] finds a trend toward a higher mean hematocrit with increasing family income within the

TABLE 8 Nutrition Surveys Comparing Number, Percent Deficient, and Percent Deficient and Low Hemoglobin, by Ethnic Group, in 10 States and New York City, 1968–1970 (Preliminary)[a]

Area	White Number	White Deficient (%)	White Deficient and Low (%)	Negro Number	Negro Deficient (%)	Negro Deficient and Low (%)	Spanish American Number	Spanish American Deficient (%)	Spanish American Deficient and Low (%)	Oriental Number	Oriental Deficient (%)	Oriental Deficient and Low (%)	American Indian Number	American Indian Deficient (%)	American Indian Deficient and Low (%)
Texas	364	N.A.[b]	8.8	1,185	N.A.	20.8	1,702	N.A.	20.2	–	–	–	–	–	–
Louisiana	1,386	N.A.	29.9	2,959	N.A.	42.3	–	–	–	–	–	–	–	–	–
New York State	2,261	1.1	8.0	462	3.7	21.7	62	1.6	16.1	–	–	–	–	–	–
Kentucky	948	3.9	16.6	308	3.6	26.7	–	–	–	–	–	–	–	–	–
Michigan	1,008	0.6	8.4	888	3.4	30.1	–	–	–	–	–	–	–	–	–
New York City	235	1.7	9.4	831	3.0	22.9	800	2.3	13.2	19	0.0	10.5	–	–	–
West Virginia	1,158	1.2	12.3	134	3.7	15.6	–	–	–	–	–	–	–	–	–
California	2,090	1.1	7.8	715	4.1	20.9	1,653	1.0	8.6	239	1.3	10.5	87	1.1	17.2
Washington	1,638	0.6	6.4	61	0.0	32.8	24	0.0	0.0	27	3.7	14.8	298	1.7	18.5
South Carolina	174	2.9	19.0	3,559	8.3	37.9	–	–	–	–	–	–	–	–	–
Massachusetts	2,957	1.0	7.2	389	3.1	20.7	180	3.4	15.1	13	0.0	0.0	–	–	–
Total	14,219	1.2	10.9	11,491	5.8	32.7	4,695	1.6	14.6	298	1.4	10.4	385	1.6	18.2

[a]For standards used in these surveys, see Table 4.
[b]N.A.–Not available
Source: Center for Disease Control.[31]

black population; this trend, however, is not exhibited in whites. Owen et al.,[54] in a study of 500 Mississippi children 1–6 years old, find a significant relation between income level and anemia: Mild anemia due to iron deficiency is especially common among the poor; 24 percent of the children in this low-income group (under $500 annual per capita income) have hemoglobin values less than 10 g/100 ml. In contrast, only 12 percent of the children from higher-income families are considered to be anemic.

The National Nutrition Survey[29] employed the Poverty Index Ratio (Orshansky Index) to separate those above and below the poverty level. This index is based on income, family size, farm or nonfarm status, and sex and age of head of household. In every surveyed state as well as in New York City, those persons below the poverty level have a higher rate of deficient hemoglobin levels than those above the poverty level (Figure 1).

Hillman and Smith[33] find low hemoglobin levels to be significantly more common in welfare families than in those not obtaining public assistance. Furthermore, this relationship persists when the data are controlled for ethnicity, as reported by Danneker[40] in a study on hemoglobin levels for 342 children 6 months to 3 years old in Allegheny County, Pennsylvania. Within the black population, the prevalence rates for anemia are the highest for those receiving public assistance: Only 19 percent of the total black sample are considered anemic (hemoglobin 10 g/100 ml or less), whereas 41.2 percent of the blacks receiving public assistance are found to have a comparable low hemoglobin concentration. Unfortunately, the sample size of the white population included in this study is too small to yield meaningful data.

Danneker also devised a crude social class index combining occupation and education of the father. Based on these criteria, 95.7 percent of the children examined are reported to be in the lowest two of five social classes. Among the black children in social class 5, 23.8 percent have hemoglobin levels under 10 g/100 ml. In contrast, the black children in social class 4 have a prevalence of 7.5 percent.

McDonough[45] compares hematocrits in white and black adults (age 45–74 years) of varying social class. Social class was based on a scale consisting of occupation, source of income, and educational attainment of head of household. High and low social classes are defined as the division of the social class scale that most nearly divides the population at its median. This division is done separately for each race, and the mean hematocrit is calculated by social class for four race–sex

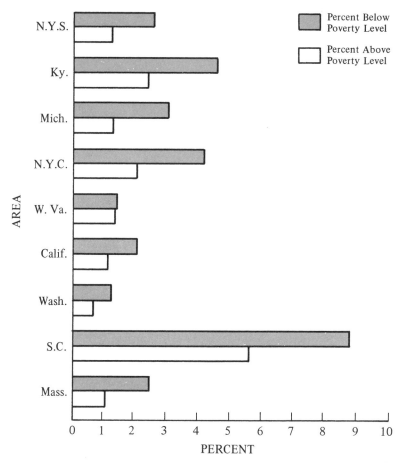

FIGURE 1 Percent of persons below and above the poverty level with deficient hemoglobin, as shown by nutrition surveys in 10 states and New York City, 1968–1970 (preliminary). From Center for Disease Control.[29]

groups. None of the social class differences within each race–sex group is found to be significant. McDonough noted, however, that only 5 percent of the black upper-class males in the study fall within the same social status scale interval as 50 percent of the upper-class white males. Thus, this measure of social class has different meanings for white and black populations and interracial comparisons are not appropriate. The explanation for the absence of a relationship between social class and hematocrit in this study may be due to the limited range of social class within this population.

Conflicting reports document lower anemia rates among private than service hospitalized patients.[20, 55, 56] In a retrospective survey among infants admitted to Columbus Children's Hospital,[56] the frequency of anemia is twice as high among service admissions than private patients using the criterion of a hemoglobin value <9.9 g/100 ml. Andelman and Sered[58] report that 76 percent of 337 infants studied in Child Welfare Stations in Chicago's Eighth District developed anemia by age 1. In contrast, Beal and Myers[59] report that out of 60 1-year-old children cared for by pediatricians in private practice in Denver, Colorado, only one had a hemoglobin value under 10 g/100 ml.

These fragmentary data are based on population samples that are often biased and poorly defined, as are the measures of social class. Nevertheless, when the extremes of the social class spectrum are compared, socioeconomic status appears to be an important variable; i.e., status is inversely related to the prevalence of anemia.

OTHER FACTORS

Pregnancy   Anemia is the most common complication of pregnancy,[5] and over 90 percent of the disease is thought to be due to iron deficiency.[5, 60-64] Studies of pregnant women all report extremely high rates of decreased hemoglobin and hematocrit values in women not receiving prophylactic iron treatment. Lund[65] reports on 4,015 maternity patients and finds 50 percent with hemoglobin levels under 11 g/100 ml. Hunter reports an overall incidence of anemia (hemoglobin 11 g/100 ml or less) of 20 percent for 4,744 patients admitted to the obstetric service of Indiana University Medical Center.[5]   As studied by Holly,[62] two thirds of the pregnant patients not receiving iron supplement develop hemoglobin values under 12 g/100 ml. Thirty-eight percent of pregnant women from low-income families in New York studied by Hillman and Smith,[53] develop hemoglobin values less than 10 g/100 ml. In a study by McGanity *et al.*,[66] 10 percent of the women in their third trimester of pregnancy have hemoglobin concentrations below 10 g/100 ml, 28 percent under 11 g/100 ml, and 57 percent had values less than 12 g/100 ml.

Birthweight and Other Associated Variables   Most investigators agree that there is an inverse relationship between birthweight and prevalence of iron deficiency in infants,[9, 20, 55, 67] which continues throughout the first 2 years of life. The latter trend is documented in Fomon and Weckwerth's[68] study of 9,986 children with birthweights over

2,500 g, and 1,709 weighing 2,500 g or less. Table 9 shows that 11.1 percent of low birthweight 2-year-olds had hemoglobin concentrations of less than 8 g/100 ml compared to 5.7 percent of their mature counterparts. These differences are not as marked in the 3-year-olds and disappear in the older children.

In addition to birthweight, parity, birth order, and spacing of pregnancies appear to be related to the development of anemia in the infant.[21, 69] It is difficult to interpret the meaning of these pregnancy-related variables because interrelations between these factors and sociodemographic variables are complex. Thus, the confounding of race, socioeconomic status, and quality and quantity of medical care with parity, birth order, and spacing of pregnancy make it especially difficult to separate independent from intervening variables.

FUNCTIONAL IMPACT

The complications of severe, chronic anemia of various etiologies are well documented.[70, 71] The most significant impact is on the cardiovascular system, which includes abnormalities in renal blood flow, increased cardiac output, alterations in venous pressure, and peripheral vascular resistance and congestive heart failure. At present in the United States these complications are relatively rare in persons with iron deficiency.[72]

TABLE 9 Summary of Concentrations of Hemoglobin Less Than 11 g/100 ml among Children Registered in Child and Youth Projects, March and April 1968

Age (years)	Birthweight > 2,500 g					Birthweight ⩽ 2,500 g				
	Number of Children	Percent of Children with Conc. Hb (g/100 ml)				Number of Children	Percent of Children with Conc. Hb (g/100 ml)			
		<11.0	<10.0	<9.0	<8.0		<11.0	<10.0	<9.0	<8.0
0.00–0.49	1,402	35.4	11.6	2.4	0.5	261	47.5	24.1	9.2	1.5
0.50–0.99	1,005	48.0	19.7	8.4	2.7	232	53.0	29.3	14.7	6.0
1.00–1.99	1,431	50.7	26.5	12.7	5.7	268	58.2	38.8	21.2	11.1
2.00–2.99	973	27.7	9.7	3.1	0.7	181	30.4	8.3	2.8	1.7
3.00–3.99	814	17.0	3.1	1.1	0.5	131	19.8	3.1	1.5	1.5
4.00–8.99	2,863	11.8	1.9	0.9	0.6	442	10.6	2.0	0.9	0.2
9.00–12.99	1,498	5.8	1.0	0.4	0.3	194	5.7	1.0	0.5	0.0

Source: Fomon and Weckwerth.[68]

For the purposes of this health evaluation program, one is particularly concerned with the effects of mild and moderate iron deficiency on child growth and development. It is very difficult to be certain that symptoms often attributed to anemia (apathy, listlessness, lassitude, somnolence, fatigue, and irritability) are indeed caused by mild iron-deficiency anemia. The effects of iron-deficiency anemia on attentiveness and learning ability were investigated by Howell.[72, 73] In children with iron-deficiency anemia (hemoglobin 9–10.5 g/100 ml) and reportedly normal IQ, the following preliminary findings are reported: "marked decreased attentiveness, more aimless manipulation, less complex and purposeful activity, narrower attention span. . .."[72] When the iron deficiency is corrected, the pattern of attentiveness and learning improved.[73] These findings are in general agreement with similar studies reported by Sulzer.[74]

Iron-deficiency anemia is now considered by many hematologists and nutritionists merely one symptom of a general nutritional/environmental health problem. One manifestation of the systemic nature of this disorder has been studied in animals by Dallman and Schwartz.[75] They document, in iron-deficient rats, diminished concentration of cytochromes and other heme proteins in cellular systems of many tissues. Some of these abnormalities respond to supplemental iron administered orally.

Although in the past it has often been stated[76] that iron-deficient persons are more susceptible to infection than iron-supplemented and well-nourished populations, recent studies[73] challenge these data. The concensus now is that increased infection rates are not associated with iron deficiency.

The effects of mild iron deficiency on growth are not well understood. For many years the classic description of the infant with iron-deficiency anemia was fat, pale, and flabby,[77] with normal height and weight.[78] Judisch, Naiman, and Oski[79] review data on 156 full-term children with nutritional iron deficiency and find that 67 percent ranked below the fiftieth percentile in body weight. Treatment with iron in a selected group resulted in accelerated weight gain. As presented at the Ross Conference,[73] the work of Hunter and Schubert does not confirm these findings. These investigators suggest that only when iron deficiency becomes so severe as to cause anorexia and a reduction in caloric intake is growth retarded. As with other effects discussed in this section, it would appear that the association of growth and mild iron deficiency requires further investigation.

REFERENCES

1. Charlton R, Bothwell T: Iron deficiency anemia. Semin Hematol 7:67–85, 1970
2. Committee on Iron Deficiency, NAS Council on Foods and Nutrition: Iron deficiency in the United States. JAMA 203:407–412, 1968
3. Finch CA: Iron deficiency anemia. Am J Clin Nutr 22:512–517, 1969
4. Gendel BR: Iron deficiency anemia. J Miss Med Assoc 1:39–42, 1960
5. Shulman I: Iron requirements in infancy. JAMA 175:118–123, 1961
6. Smith N, Rosello S: Iron deficiency in infancy and childhood. J Clin Nutr 1:275–286, 1953
7. Statement by Committee on Nutrition of the American Academy of Pediatrics. Newsletter, American Academy of Pediatrics (Suppl), December 15, 1970.
8. Hunter CA: Iron deficiency anemia in pregnancy. Surg Gynecol Obstet 110:210–214, 1960
9. Woodruff C: Nutritional anemias in early childhood. Am J Clin Nutr 22:504–511, 1969
10. Wintrobe MM: Clinical Hematology. Philadelphia, Lea & Febiger, 1967
11. Shils ME, Sass M, Goldwater LJ: A microhematocrit method and its evaluation. Am J Clin Pathol 22:157, 1955
12. McInroy RA: A microhematocrit for determining the pack cell volume and hemoglobin concentration on capillary blood. J Clin Pathol 7 (No 1):32–36, 1954
13. Kaucher M, Moyer EZ, Harrison AP, et al: Nutritional status of children. VII. Hemoglobin. Am Diet Assoc J 24:496–502, 1948
14. Eppright ES, Marlatt AL, Patton MB, et al: Nutritional status of 9- 10-and 11-year-old public school children in Iowa, Kansas, and Ohio: 11 blood findings. Wooster, Ohio, Ohio Agric Exp Stn (Res Bull 794) 1957
15. Morgan AF: Nutritional Status USA Calif Agric Ext Stn Bull 769, 1959
16. Pearson HA: Iron requirements and recommended intakes, Iron Nutrition in Infancy. Report of the 62nd Ross Conference on Pediatric Research, Columbus, Ohio, Ross Laboratories, 1970
17. Maternal and Child Health Service: Comments regarding the March–April children and youth survey, 1968. Washington, DC, Department of Health, Education, and Welfare, 1969
18. Adams M, Scott R: Iron-deficiency anemia in Negro infants and children in the metropolitan area of the District of Columbia. Med Ann DC 32:391–393, 1963
19. Burroughs PH, Huenemann RL: Iron deficiency in rural infants and children. J Am Diet Assoc 57:122–128, 1970
20. Fomon SJ: Prevention of iron deficiency anemia in infants and children of preschool age. Washington, DC, Government Printing Office, 1970.(PHS Publication No 2085).
21. Guest GM, Brown EW: Erythrocytes and hemoglobin of the blood in infancy and childhood. III. Factors in variability, statistical studies. Am J Dis Child 93:486–509, 1957

22. Gutelius M: The problem of iron deficiency anemia in the preschool Negro child. Am J Public Health 59:290–295, 1969
23. Haughton J: Nutritional anemia of infancy and childhood. Am J Public Health 53:1121–1126, 1963
24. Lahey M: Iron deficiency anemia. Pediatr Clin N Am 93:481–496, 1957
25. Pearson HA: Anemia in preschool children in the United States of America. Pediatr Res 1:169–172, 1967
26. Pearson HA: Iron requirements and recommended intakes, Iron Nutrition in Infancy. Report of the 62nd Ross Conference on Pediatric Research, Columbus, Ohio, Ross Laboratories, 1970
27. Mugrage E, Anderson M: Red blood cell values in adolescents. Am J Dis Child 55:776–783, 1938
28. National Center for Health Statistics: Mean Blood Hematocrit of Adults, United States 1960–1962. Department of Health, Education, and Welfare, Washington, DC, Government Printing Office, 1967 (PHS Publication No 1000, Series 11, No 24)
29. Center for Disease Control: Ten State Nutrition Survey in the United States, 1968–1970, Preliminary Report to the Congress. Department of Health, Education, and Welfare, Public Health Service, Health Services and Mental Health Administration, Atlanta, 1971
30. Daniel W, Rowland A: Hemoglobin and hematocrit values of adolescents— Nutritional survey of low income groups. Clin Pediatr 8:181–184, 1969
31. Heald F: Iron deficiency anemia in adolescent girls. Postgrad Med 27:104–108, 1960
32. Moench L: The incidence and significance of anemia in an unselected group of "well" individuals. Proc Life Ext Exam 2:133–139, 1940
33. Odland L, Ostle R: Clinical and biochemical studies of Montana adolescents. J Am Diet Assoc 32: 823–828, 1956
34. Verghese KP, Ferebee DB, Ferguson AD, et al: Studies in growth and development. XI Hemoglobin concentration in adolescents. J Pediatr 67:1194–1196, 1965
35. Williams HH, Parker JS, Pierce ZH, et al: Nutritional status survey, Groton Township, New York. J Am Diet Assoc 27:215–221, 1951
36. Kirschenfeld M, Tew H: Prevalence and significance of anemia as seen in a rural general practice. JAMA 158:807–811, 1955
37. Munday B, Shepherd ML, Emerson L, et al: Hemoglobin differences in healthy white and Negro infants. Am J Dis Child 55:776–783, 1938
38. Milam D, Muench H: Hemoglobin levels in specific race, age, and sex groups of a normal North Carolina population. J Lab Clin Med 31:878–885, 1946
39. Christakis G, Miridjanian A, Nath L, et al: A nutritional epidemiologic investigation of 642 New York City children. Am J Clin Nutr 21:107–126, 1968
40. Danneker D: Anemia in selected Allegheny County child health conference populations. Pittsburgh, Allegheny Health Dept, 1966
41. Hutcheson RH: Iron deficiency anemia in Tennessee among rural poor children. Public Health Rep 83:939–943, 1968
42. Hutcheson RH: Iron deficiency as a public health problem, Iron Nutrition in Infancy. Report of the 62nd Ross Conference on Pediatric Research, Columbus, Ohio, Ross Laboratories, 1970

43. Myers M, Mable JA, Stare FJ: A nutrition study of school children in a depressed urban district. J Am Diet Assoc 53:234–242, 1968
44. Zee P, Walters T, Mitchell C: Nutrition and poverty in preschool children. JAMA 213:739–742, 1970
45. McDonough JR, Hames CG, Garrison GE, et al: The relations of hematocrit to cardiovascular states of health in the Negro and white population of Evans County, Georgia. J Chronic Dis 18:243–257, 1965
46. Bradfield R, Brun T: Nutritional status of California Mexican-Americans. Am J Clin Nutr 23:798–806, 1970
47. Corbett T: Iron deficiency anemia in a Pueblo Indian Village. JAMA 205:186, 1968
48. Lantz E, Wood P: Nutrition of New Mexican Spanish-American and "Anglo" adolescents. J Am Diet Assoc 34:145–153, 1958
49. Lantz E, Wood P: Nutritional condition of New Mexican children. J Am Diet Assoc 34:1199–1207, 1958
50. Perkins GB, Church GM: Report of pediatric evaluations of a sample of Indian children on Wind River Indian Reservation, 1957. Am J Public Health 50:181–189, 1960
51. Interdepartmental Committee on Nutrition for National Defense and Division of Indian Health, United States Public Health Service: Blackfeet Indian Reservation Nutrition Survey, Washington, DC, Department of Health, Education, and Welfare, 1964
52. Interdepartmental Committee on Nutrition for National Defense and Division of Indian Health, United States Public Health Service: Fort Belknap Indian Reservation Nutrition Survey, Washington, DC, Department of Health, Education, and Welfare, 1964
53. Hillman RW, Smith HS: Hemoglobin patterns in low-income families. Public Health Rep 83:61–67, 1968
54. Owen GM, Garry PJ, Kram KM, et al: Nutritional status of Mississippi preschool children. Am J Clin Nutr 22:1444–1458, 1969
55. Fomon SJ: Infant Nutrition. Philadelphia, WB Saunders Co, 1967
56. Kripke S, Sanders E: Prevalence of iron-deficiency anemia among infants and young children seen at rural ambulatory clinics. Am J Clin Nutr 23:716–724, 1970
57. Shaw R, Robertson WO: Anemia among hospitalized infants. Ohio State Med J 60:45–47, 1964
58. Andelman M, Sered B: Utilization of dietary iron by term infants. Am J Dis Child 3:45–55, 1966
59. Beal VA, Myers AJ: Iron nutriture from infancy to adolescence. Am J Public Health 60:666–678, 1970
60. Henderson PA: Anemia of pregnancy. Obstet Gynecol 24:752–756, 1964
61. Holly RG: Anemia in pregnancy. Clin Obstet Gynecol 1:15–40, 1958
62. Holly RG: Anemia in pregnancy. Obstet Gynecol 5:562–568, 1955
63. Hood WE: Iron deficiency anemia in pregnancy. South Med J 56:170–172, 1963
64. Lowenstein L, Hsieh Y, Brunton L, et al: Nutritional deficiency and anemia in pregnancy. Postgrad Med 31:72–78, 1962
65. Lund CJ: Studies on the iron deficiency anemia of pregnancy, including plasma volume, total hemoglobin, erythrocyte protoporphyrin in treated and

untreated normal and anemic patients. Am J Obstet Gynecol 62:947–963, 1951

66. McGanity WJ, Bridgeforth EB, Darby WJ: Vanderbilt cooperative study of maternal and infant nutrition. JAMA 168:2138–2145, 1958

67. Diamond LK: Nutritional anemia in infants and children. Postgrad Med 34:238–243, 1963

68. Fomon SJ, Weckwerth VE: Hemoglobin Concentrations of Children Registered for Care in C&Y Projects during March and April 1968. (mimeographed) Department of Pediatrics, University of Iowa and Systems Development Project, University of Minnesota

69. Jacobs I: Iron deficiency anemia in infancy and childhood. Gen Pract 21:93–97, 1960

70. Bradley SE, Bradley GP: Renal function during chronic anemia in men. Blood 2:192–202, 1947

71. Whitaker W: Some effects of severe chronic anemia on the circulatory system. Q J Med 25:175–183, 1956

72. Howell DA: Significance of Iron Deficiency: Consequences of Mild Deficiency in Children. Presented at Food and Nutrition Board Workshop Conference. The Extent and Meanings of Nutritional Iron-Deficiency in the United States. (mimeographed) Washington, DC, National Academy of Sciences, March 8–9, 1971

73. Iron Nutrition in Infancy. Report of the 62nd Ross Conference on Pediatric Research, Ross Laboratories, Columbus, Ohio, 1970

74. Sulzer J: Significance of Iron Deficiency: Effects of Iron Deficiency on Psychological Tests in Children. Presented at Food and Nutrition Board Workshop Conference. The Extent and Meaning of Nutritional Iron Deficiency in the United States. (mimeographed) Washington, DC, National Academy of Sciences, March 8–9, 1971

75. Dallman P, Schwartz H: Distribution of cytochrome c in myoglobin in rats with dietary iron deficiency. Pediatrics 35:677–685, 1965

76. MacKay HMM: Nutritional Anemia in Infancy with Special Reference to Iron Deficiency. Medical Research Council. London, HM Stationery Office, 1931. (Special Report Series No 157). p. 96

77. Githens JH, Hathaway WE: Iron deficiency anemia of infants. Clin Pediatr 2:477, 1959

78. Nelson WE: Textbook of Pediatrics. Philadelphia, WB Saunders Co, 1964, p 1018

79. Judisch JM, Naiman JL, Oski FA: The fallacy of the fat iron deficient child. Pediatrics 37:987–990, 1966

BIBLIOGRAPHY

AMA Council on Drugs: AMA Drug Evaluation, 1971. Chicago, American Medical Association, 1971

Committee on Nutrition of the American Academy of Pediatrics: Statement. Newsletter, American Academy of Pediatrics (Suppl), December 15, 1970

Iron-Fortified Formulas for Infants. The Medical Letter 13:65–66, 1971

FIVE

Essential Hypertension

SUMMARY

An adequate evaluation of the patient with an elevated blood pressure will reflect not only the quality of the general history and physical examination but, specifically, those aspects related to the cardiovascular system. It will provide an opportunity to assess the appropriate use of laboratory tests and will reveal much about the manner in which drugs are used. The proper management of hypertension requires careful and long-term follow-up and its assessment will bring forth data on the control of diet and psychologic problems. In addition, this tracer provides an opportunity to evaluate the appropriate use of inpatient facilities both for the diagnosis of a complex chronic vascular disease and for treatment of the complications associated with hypertension.

CLASSIFICATION

Essential hypertension can be broadly defined as a sustained elevation of blood pressure without evident cause. There is much controversy as to the definitions of "sustained," "elevated," and "without evident cause." Substantial evidence exists, however, to support the opinion that essential hypertension is a quantitative and not a qualitative disease; that is, the distribution of blood pressures on the far right of the curve represents a quantitative deviation from "statistically usual" pressures. (For a detailed discussion of the quantitative–qualitative debate see References 1–5.) In light of the present controversy, the epidemiology of essential hypertension has been reviewed within the context of the distribution of blood pressure in defined populations.

EPIDEMIOLOGY

Age and Sex   Recent blood pressure surveys in the United States have provided much evidence that pressure levels are positively related to age. Young white females, in general, have lower mean systolic pressure than males, with a reversal of this sex pattern in older age groups. An increase in mean diastolic pressure with age is reported in most cross-sectional population studies. There are conflicting data regarding the relationship of sex to mean diastolic pressure.

Race   There are many reports that document the higher mean pressures and higher prevalence of elevated pressure among black Americans than among age- and sex-matched white Americans. In five biracial studies, the black–white differences are found at all ages and in both sexes with a smaller difference for diastolic, rather than systolic, pressure and for younger, rather than older, age groups. A tabulation of racial–regional differences in mean blood pressure throughout the world documents widespread interracial variation. Although the data are not conclusive, there is much information to suggest that intraracial differences in blood pressure are greater than interracial ones and that much of the interracial differences can be explained by environmental variables.

Socioeconomic Status   Data on the occupational dimension of socioeconomic status is inconsistent. There is some evidence for an inverse relationship between physical activity and blood pressure, but it is unconvincing. In general, variations in amount of habitual physical exercise are insufficient to explain differences in blood pressure. Studies of both white and black American populations show educational status and pressure to be inversely related. A similar relationship holds for family income for blacks below $7,000 per year, but not for the white population.

Other Factors   Body build and body bulk measures are directly related to blood pressure levels. Although there are many problems in the interpretation of data on body build, weight-related factors appear to be most important; this trend is apparent in whites, in females, and in middle-aged adults. Dietary factors also may be directly related to blood pressure variation; apparently the level of sodium intake is the most important of these. Although there is some conflict about the role of sodium, it is felt by several to be a critical dietary factor.

FUNCTIONAL IMPACT

Essential hypertension, in contrast to secondary hypertension caused by adrenal, renal, or specific vascular lesions, usually has its onset between 35 and 45 years of age. Many symptoms commonly associated with hypertension, such as headache and vertigo, have not been studied carefully in a controlled manner, and it is not clear whether they occur more frequently in hypertensive than in nonhypertensive subjects. Long-term follow-up studies (greater than 10 years) however, document that between 50 and 70 percent of patients with essential hypertension develop an enlarged heart and that a similar percent develop symptoms of heart failure. Detailed studies by the Society of Actuaries show that men with a casual blood pressure of 140 mmHg systolic and 90 mmHg diastolic, and free of other impairments, are subject to about 50 percent increased mortality as compared with the average of all insured lives. This risk increases to 100 percent when the blood pressure is 145/95 and to 200 percent when the blood pressure reaches 160/100. The usual causes of death associated with hypertension are heart disease, cerebral vascular disease, and renal failure. It is clear that the treatment of malignant hypertension improves the patient's prognosis by reducing the chances of death from stroke and renal failure, but not from myocardial infarction. Patients with moderate hypertension (diastolic pressure 115–129 mmHg) have been shown clearly to benefit from antihypertensive treatment. The effect is due to a reduction in cardiovascular deaths and nonfatal cardiovascular episodes; as with malignant hypertension, however, the incidence of myocardial infarction remained unchanged. Although there is controversy over the impact of treatment of mild hypertension (diastolic pressure 90–114 mmHg), the Veterans Administration Cooperative Study indicates that treatment reduces morbidity, as well as mortality. Freis has reported that treatment is effective in reducing morbidity in patients with mean diastolic blood pressures as low as 105 mmHg.

A MINIMAL-CARE PLAN FOR HYPERTENSION*

I. Screening

A. *Method.* The systolic pressure is recorded at the onset of the first Korotkoff sound and the diastolic at the final disappearance of the second or the change if the sound persists.

B. *Criteria.* An individual is judged in need of evaluation for elevated blood pressure if the mean of three or more systolic or diastolic pressures exceeds the age-specific criteria specified below:

Males and Females	Systolic (mmHg)	Diastolic (mmHg)
18–44 years	140	90
45–64 years	150	95
65 years or older	160	95

II. Evaluation

In the evaluation of elevated blood pressure, the history and physical-examination data listed below should be obtained early in the evaluation.

A. *History.* (1) Personal and social history; (2) family history of high blood pressure, coronary artery disease, or stroke; (3) previous diagnosis of high blood pressure (females: toxemia of pregnancy or pre-eclampsia) and time of first occurence; (4) previous treatment for high blood pressure: when started, when stopped, and drugs used; (5) chest pain, pressure, or tightness—location, length of symptoms, frequency of symptoms, effect of deep breathing, description of feeling (crushing, strangling, smothering), symptom temporarily curtails activity, and pain radiates into left shoulder, arm, or jaw and is accompanied by nausea, shortness of breath, and/or fast or fluttering heart beat; (6) feet swell; (7) shortness of breath; (8) awakens wheezing or feeling smothered or choked; (9) sleeps on two or more pillows; (10) prior history of kidney trouble, nephrosis, or nephritis; (11) history of kidney infection, and (12) prior x-ray examination of kidneys.

B. *Physical examination.* (1) Weight and height; (2) blood pressure: supine and upright; (3) funduscopic; (4) heart: abnormal sounds or rhythm; (5) neck: thyroid and neck veins; (6) abdomen: standard description, including abdominal bruit; and (7) extremities: peripheral pulses and edema.

*From Kessner DM, Kalk CE: Assessing health quality—the case for tracers. N Engl J Med 288:191, 1973. Reprinted by permission.

C. *Laboratory.* (1) Urinalysis; (2) hematocrit or hemoglobin; and (3) blood urea nitrogen or serum creatinine.

D. *Other tests.* (1) Electrocardiogram; and (2) rapid sequence intravenous pyelogram (IVP), if the patient is less than 30 years of age or if diastolic is 130 mmHg or greater.

III. Diagnosis

A. *Essential hypertension.* As described above under I. B. *Criteria,* provided there is no evidence of secondary hypertension.

B. *Secondary hypertension.* Hypertension secondary to renal, adrenal, thyroid, or primary vascular disease.

IV. Management

All drugs are prescribed in acceptable dosages adjusted to the individual patient, contraindications are observed, and patients are monitored for common side effects according to information detailed in *AMA Drug Evaluations, 1971.* Fixed-dosage combinations should not be used for initial therapy.

A. *Mild essential hypertension (diastolic pressure of 115 mmHg).* (1) Initial treatment with thiazides alone in a diuretic dose; (2) if pressure is not reduced by 10 mmHg or to lowest level that patient can tolerate without symptoms of hypotension in 2 to 4 weeks, add one of the following to thiazide: alpha methyldopa, reserpine, or hydralazine.

B. *Moderate essential hypertension (diastolic pressure of 115 to 130 mmHg).* (1) Initial treatment with thiazide and alpha methyldopa, reserpine, or hydralazine; (2) if no response after 2 to 4 weeks, change to thiazide–reserpine–hydralazine or thiazide–guanethidine combination.

C. *Severe essential hypertension (diastolic pressure of 130 mmHg or Keith-Wagener Grade III or IV funduscopic changes).* Refer to specialist, hospitalize, or both.

D. *Secondary hypertension.* Treat, or refer for treatment of, primary condition.

E. *Undetermined etiology or no response to treatment.* Hypertension of undetermined etiology or that does not respond to treatment regimens above requires further evaluation, to include (1) serum sodium and potassium, and (2) rapid sequence IVP, if not previously performed.

EPIDEMIOLOGY

The commonly accepted definition of essential hypertension can be summarized as a sustained elevation of both systolic and diastolic blood pressure without evident cause. Attempts to define operationally the key elements of this condition—"sustained," "elevated," and "without evident cause"— have been inconsistent and difficult to implement. Moreover, there is a body of evidence to support the opinion that essential hypertension is a quantitative and not a qualitative disease; that is, the upper end of a blood pressure distribution curve represents a quantitative deviation from "statistically usual" pressures.* Hence, most recent epidemiologic work, giving cognizance to the quantitative hypothesis, has investigated the epidemiology of essential hypertension within the context of the epidemiology of blood pressure.

The rationale for this approach to the study of essential hypertension, which will be followed in this review, follows:[1, 3]

1. The study of blood pressure distributions in defined populations gives no indication of a natural division into normal and diseased groups; i.e., distributions are characteristically continuous and unimodal.

2. Cases of secondary hypertension (e.g., elevations of pressure secondary to primary hyperaldosteronism, Cushings' syndrome, chronic renal disease, and renal vascular disease) form an insignificant portion of the "hypertensive" populations.

3. Casual blood pressure measurements alone are prognostic of future morbidity and mortality from cardiovascular lesions.

4. Even if blood pressure measurements are eventually shown to be incomplete diagnostic information for the identification of essential hypertensives, knowledge of the factors influencing blood pressure regulation and associated with blood pressure elevations, which can be gathered through this approach, will inevitably help clarify the etiology of essential hypertension.

While the relative merits of considering the epidemiology of essential hypertension within the context of the epidemiology of blood pressure are clear, this approach produces many difficulties. Blood pressure measurements are subject to considerable actual and ob-

---

*For discussions of the quantitative–qualitative debate, see References 1–5.

served variation. The ramifications of these variations for epidemiologic study are important, but a detailed consideration of these factors is outside the scope of this review. Pertinent variables that are sources of error include diurnal variation, casual versus basal pressures, and observer and technical biases.[3, 6-12]

It must be emphasized that these sources of error call into question the validity, accuracy, and precision of blood pressure measurements. It thus becomes mandatory that in epidemiologic studies the inherent instability of the measurements be balanced by careful controls and standardization of procedures.

It is understood that a literature review cannot reconcile all methodologic incompatibilities. In order to eliminate much artifactual variation, this review concentrates on the most recent surveys that describe pressures on representative samples or total communities, utilize standardized procedures (including observer training and control for observer variability), and, in general, take more than one pressure reading.

AGE AND SEX

Age- and sex-related trends in blood pressure are well documented. The consensus of reports from prevalence studies* conducted on all but certain primitive populations documents (a) definite age and sex trends in mean blood pressure, with young women having lower mean pressures than young men and the reverse in the older age groups, and (b) distributions showing a displacement of pressures toward higher values with increasing age.

Mean Pressures—Systolic Several recent large-scale studies report that young females have lower mean systolic pressures than young males, with the reverse situation occuring at older ages.[6, 14-17] Two studies of biracial southern populations report exceptions to this trend, with mean blood pressures among Negro females consistently higher than Negro males from early adulthood (see Race, p. 135).[18, 19] There is less consensus on the age range in which this crossover occurs. McDonough *et al.*[18] report higher rates for females around age 35 in a southern white sample, as do Boyle *et al.*[19] in a similar black population. Many

---

*This report focuses on published material reporting blood pressure in *adult* populations. The age pattern generally documented in children describes a sharp rise in the first 2 years of life, with the rate of increase slowing until a second sharp spurt at puberty.[13,14]

investigations of white populations in Europe and the United States document this sex pattern a decade later.[14, 15, 20-22] The National Health Examination Survey,[6] based on a nationwide probability sample, finds mean female pressures not exceeding those of males until the 55–64-year age group; similar results come from a recent biracial study conducted in California[23] and a large-scale survey in Hiroshima.[24]

The rate of increase of mean systolic blood pressure by age, taken from an analysis of four pressure surveys,[6] is shown in Figure 1. National prevalence data suggest that the rate of increase in systolic pressure becomes greater the older the person is, with the exception of females over 70 years.[6] This is in contrast to data from Bergen, Norway, that show the rate rising until age 60 in men and 50 in women, after which it falls.[22] The Framingham data[15] (while restricted in age range) also show a fall in rate of increase around age 50 that is much more pronounced than in the Bergen data.

Mean Pressures—Diastolic Although less striking than trends found for mean systolic pressure, an increase in mean diastolic pressure with age is reported in most cross-sectional data. Studies of Japanese and Chinese samples, however, as well as of biracial populations from Georgia and the Bahamas, document no sex trend.[17,18,24,25] The Charleston study[19] shows a sex crossover among their white population sample, while among blacks, females maintain higher pressures at most ages. In contrast, data on a large biracial sample from Alameda County[23] documents no sex pattern among blacks; among whites, mean diastolic pressure of males, however, is consistently higher than females over the entire age range studied. Several studies[15, 20, 22] of white populations indicate a sex crossover similar to that observed with mean systolic pressure.

All studies are in agreement that the mean diastolic pressure curve has a different configuration than the systolic curve, with a decline in rate of rise—or an actual fall—sometime after middle age.[6, 14, 16, 18, 22, 23, 26] As can be seen in Figure 2, many investigators report a shallower gradient in mean diastolic pressure with age among men than women, with a greater tendency to plateau before middle age and to level off, or fall, a decade earlier.

The rate of increase in mean diastolic blood pressure with age is closely examined in the National Health Survey analysis.[6] It is clear from Figure 3 this decreases with age in the nationwide sample, ex-

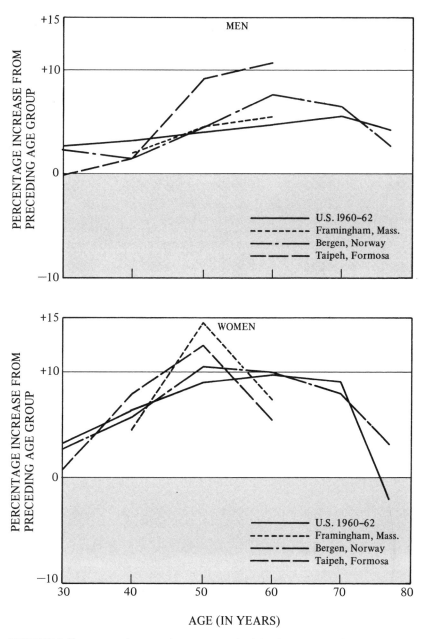

FIGURE 1 Percentage increase in mean systolic blood pressure, taken from four surveys, by sex and age. From National Center for Health Statistics.[6]

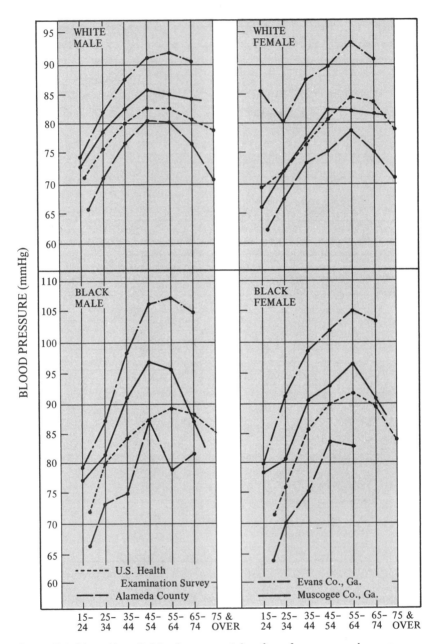

FIGURE 2 Mean diastolic blood pressure, taken from four surveys, by race, sex, and age. From Borhani and Borkman.[23]

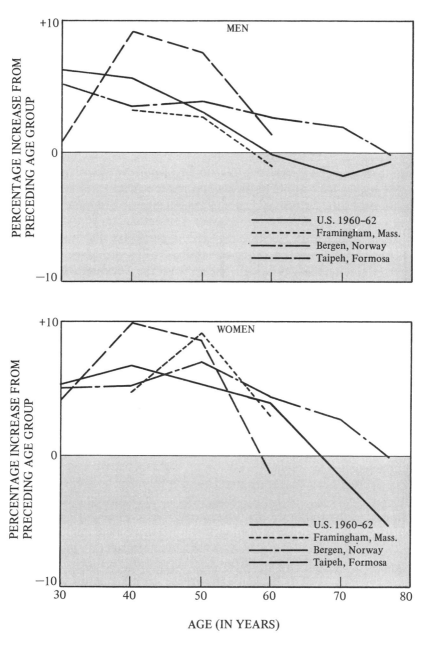

FIGURE 3 Percentage increase in mean diastolic blood pressure, taken from four surveys, by sex and age. From National Center for Health Statistics.[6]

cept in females 30–40 years old. After age 64 in men and 74 in women, the rate of change becomes negative. The Bergen data[22] show similar trends, while the Framingham study[15] reports a sharp rate of increase in pressure in the 30–50- year age group for both sexes.

Several large-scale studies have employed regression (and more recently multiple regression) analysis to estimate the significance of age to the distribution of mean blood pressure. Regression analyses have consistently shown mean blood pressure to be significantly related to age and/or age squared.[22, 26-30] Simple correlation coefficients between age and either systolic or diastolic pressures in each race–sex group of a nationwide sample, are highly significant; coefficients tend to be higher for systolic pressures and for females.[28]

Study of the Framingham and National Health Examination distributions also reveal an age–sex crossover effect similar to that observed with mean pressures. Analysis of selected percentile distributions[14, 22, 23] show age–sex trends similar to those already described (see Figures 4 and 5). The percentile curves plotted from the Tecumseh, Michigan, Bergen, Norway, and Alameda County, California, data clearly document the increased rate or rise in systolic pressure among females by age, with pressures in each percentile starting lower than the comparable male group and ending higher.[14, 22, 23] The diastolic curves show a similar, though less pronounced, age–sex trend.

Longitudinal Studies   The shortcomings of cross-sectional data for the documentation of age trends are well known: There is a tendency to understate the real rise in blood pressure with age, "since young persons with high blood pressure are less apt to survive to an older age than are young persons with low blood pressure."[6] Conversely, in cohort studies, the tendency of mean pressure to rise with age could be exaggerated because differing environmental influences might cause a selective pressure rise among older persons in any given population. Similarly, the well-documented tendency for mean blood pressure in women to exceed that of men in the upper age ranges might be due to selective mortality—the tendency for women to tolerate pressure elevations better than men.

Nearly all longitudinal studies have been conducted on selected populations (e.g., military, hospital, insured, working). As with the cross-sectional trends, these studies indicate that mean pressures rise with age. However, Stamler et al.[31] report that a subsample of their population, when followed prospectively, experienced no rise in pressure with age. In a longitudinal study of healthy males, Harlow et al.[32]

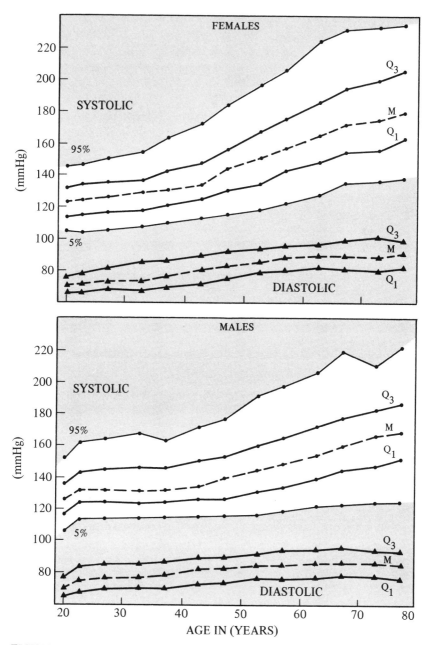

FIGURE 4 Medians and quartiles of blood pressure by sex and age in Bergen, Norway. From Boe *et al.*[22]

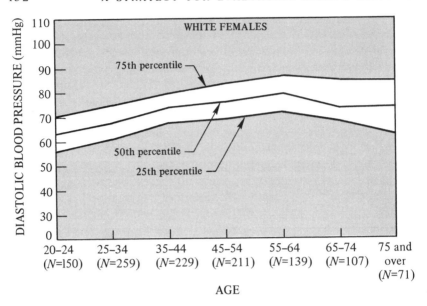

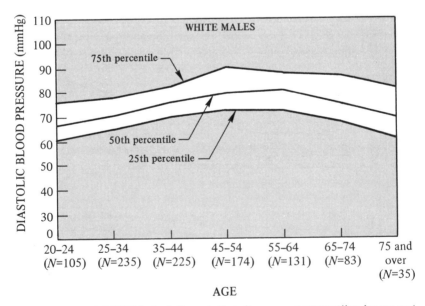

FIGURE 5 Systolic and diastolic pressure percentiles, by sex and

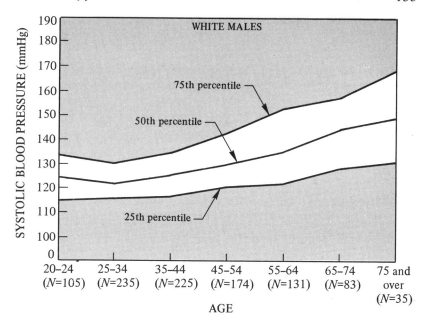

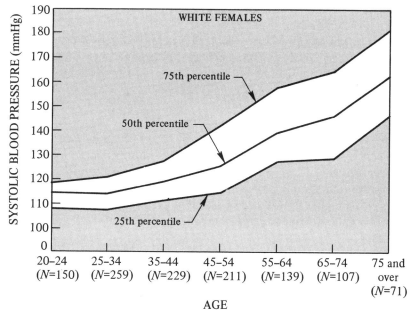

age, in Alameda County, California. From Borhani and Borkman.[23]

find that age alone did not have a significant effect on blood pressure after controlling for weight gain and a positive family history of vascular disease.

Miall and Lovell,[20] in one of the first attempts to apply multiple regression analysis to longitudinal blood pressure data, assess the relative contributions of age and pressure level in determining change in pressure with age in two South Wales populations. Over 5,000 persons in two communities were followed for 8.5 to 10 years, and the mean of the initial and final blood pressure readings were used. Results of the simple regression analysis show no pattern when change of pressure over the entire period of observation is regressed on age, while 22 of the coefficients calculated for change of pressure on mean pressure are positive and significant. The multiple regression analysis shows similar results: All but one of the significant age coefficients are negative, while all 25 mean pressure coefficients are positive and significant. The authors thus conclude that "change of pressure is related to pressure level rather than to age."

The Framingham data[13] are analyzed subsequently in an attempt to replicate the findings of Miall and Lovell. Contrary to those findings, however, Feinleib *et al.*[13] conclude "for the Framingham cohort that the tendency of blood pressure to rise as people get older is unrelated to their initial blood pressure level. The relationship between age and blood pressure remains a controversial question and indeed may vary with the populations under study."

RACE

The role of race in the determination of blood pressure level and change in level with age has been of long-standing concern for investigators throughout the world. Most pertinent to our purposes is the often-reported finding that American blacks have higher mean pressures and a higher prevalence of elevated pressures, as well as higher cardiovascular mortality rates, than age- and sex-matched American whites.[18, 33–38]

Several large-scale cross-sectional studies conducted recently in the United States have explored racial differences in blood pressure. In each of five major studies,[16, 18, 19, 23, 39] Negroes are found to have higher mean systolic and diastolic blood pressures at all ages in both sexes. Mean systolic pressure curves generally show a steeper rise in Negroes of both sexes before middle age; after middle age the mean differences between race–sex groups stabilize or decrease. In all five

United States biracial studies, the black–white difference is smaller for diastolic than systolic pressures and for younger than older age groups. There is also some indication of race–sex differences in mean pressure trends in these five studies. Whereas in each the mean systolic and diastolic pressures of white females cross those of males around middle age, two southern surveys[18, 19] fail to document this pattern in black females; they show higher mean systolic and diastolic pressures at most ages.

Blood pressure distributions from these studies also reveal consistent racial differences. All studies report an earlier and greater spread of pressures toward higher values with increasing age among blacks, resulting in less-peaked distributions than are found in age- and sex-matched white groups (Figures 6 and 7). There is thus a greater proportion of blacks of both sexes with higher pressures compared to whites (Tables 1 and 2). Some studies[18, 19, 23] also reveal distributions

TABLE 1   Number and Percent Distribution of Systolic Blood Pressures for White and Negro Adults, by Sex, in the United States, 1960–1962

| Pressure (mmHg) | No. of Persons (in thousands) | | | | Percent Distribution | | | |
| | Men | | Women | | Men | | Women | |
	White	Negro	White	Negro	White	Negro	White	Negro
Under 90	43	–	167	18	0.1	–	0.3	0.3
90–99	584	99	2,258	196	1.3	1.9	4.4	3.1
100–109	3,517	434	7,566	825	7.6	8.4	14.8	13.3
110–119	8,866	955	11,655	1,333	19.0	18.4	22.8	21.4
120–129	11,287	920	9,432	919	24.2	17.7	18.4	14.8
130–139	9,290	814	6,813	698	20.0	15.7	13.3	11.2
140–149	5,558	571	4,296	536	11.9	11.0	8.4	8.6
150–159	3,382	522	2,676	420	7.3	10.1	5.2	6.8
160–169	1,734	319	2,047	370	3.7	6.1	4.0	6.0
170–179	1,060	249	1,467	246	2.3	4.8	2.9	3.9
180–189	447	157	1,085	236	1.0	3.0	2.1	3.8
190–199	416	86	843	127	0.9	1.6	1.6	2.0
200–209	214	34	465	61	0.5	0.7	0.9	1.0
210–219	74	–	172	152	0.2	–	0.3	2.4
220–229	53	25	91	25	0.1	0.5	0.2	0.4
230–239	27	–	88	19	0.1	–	0.2	0.3
240–249	–	–	11	–	–	–	0.0	–
250–259	9	9	13	–	0.0	0.2	0.0	–
Over 260	–	–	36	36	–	–	0.1	0.6
TOTAL	46.561	5,195	51,184	6,219	100.0	100.0	100.0	100.0

Source: National Center for Health Statistics.[39]

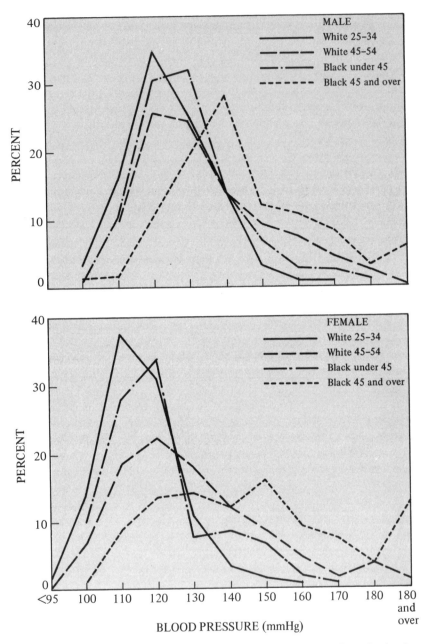

FIGURE 6 Systolic blood pressure for selected age–race groups. From Borhani and Borkman.[23]

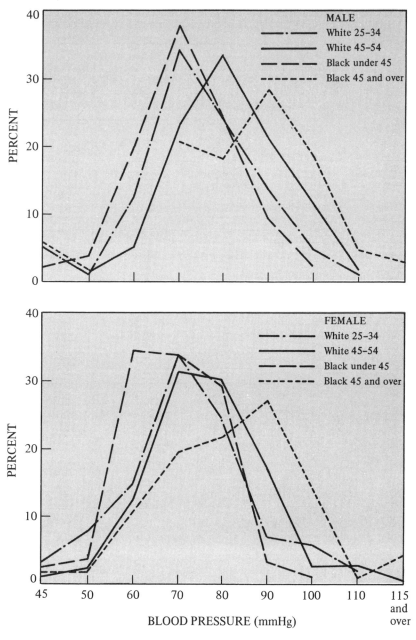

FIGURE 7 Diastolic blood pressure for selected age–race groups. From Borhani and Borkman.[23]

TABLE 2   Number and Percent Distribution of Diastolic Blood Pressures for White and Negro Adults, by Sex, in the United States, 1960–1962

Pressure (mmHg)	No. of Persons (in thousands)				Percent Distribution			
	Men		Women		Men		Women	
	White	Negro	White	Negro	White	Negro	White	Negro
Under 50	490	43	314	25	1.1	0.8	0.6	0.4
50–54	367	42	552	93	0.8	0.8	1.1	1.5
55–59	846	108	1,573	74	1.8	2.1	3.1	1.2
60–64	2,362	167	3,619	279	5.1	3.2	7.1	4.5
65–69	5,094	461	6,698	714	10.9	8.9	13.1	11.5
70–74	6,689	686	8,636	680	14.4	13.2	16.9	10.9
75–79	9,807	722	9,364	976	21.1	13.9	18.3	15.7
80–84	7,191	686	7,923	891	15.4	13.2	15.5	14.3
85–89	5,936	598	4,999	706	12.7	11.5	9.8	11.4
90–94	3,520	507	3,250	441	7.6	9.8	6.3	7.1
95–99	2,023	638	1,819	457	4.3	12.3	3.6	7.4
100–104	990	182	1,132	243	2.1	3.5	2.2	3.9
105–109	663	108	616	221	1.4	2.1	1.2	3.6
110–114	243	132	191	99	0.5	2.5	0.4	1.6
115–119	162	55	234	145	0.3	1.1	0.5	2.3
120–124	80	27	109	52	0.2	0.5	0.2	0.8
125–129	–	25	64	83	–	0.5	0.1	1.3
130–134	49	–	18	14	0.1	–	0.0	0.2
Over 135	48	9	72	24	0.1	0.2	0.1	0.4
TOTAL	46,561	5,195	51,184	6,219	100.0	100.0	100.0	100.0

Source: National Center for Health Statistics.[39]

with a greater skew to the right at most ages among blacks; this is especially marked for systolic pressure in black females.

Despite the consistency with which investigations document variation in blood pressure by race, it is important to consider the five major biracial studies used above to illustrate interracial variation in blood pressure. Mean pressure of blacks is higher and a greater interracial difference is documented in all three southern surveys[18, 19, 40] than is found in either the Alameda County[23] or the National Health Survey.[39] In the latter, the blood pressure of Negro adults on the average is greater than the pressure of white adults by 5.6 mmHg systolic and 5.0 mmHg diastolic. In contrast, the three southern surveys display interracial differences in mean pressures of approximately 15 mmHg systolic and 10 mmHg diastolic. Borhani and Borkman[23] tabulate these mean differences in age and sex groups for all the studies in question with the exception of the Charleston study (Table 3). The

TABLE 3 Number of Age–Sex Comparisons[a] (in mmHg) Difference between Negroes and Whites in Four Surveys

Difference in Mean Blood Pressure (mmHg)	Alameda County, Calif.	U.S. Health Examination Survey	Muscogee County, Ga.	Evans County, Ga.
Systolic				
<5	6	5	2	2
5.0–9.9	6	5	–	1
10.0–14.9	–	2	3	1
15.0–19.9	–	2	3	6
⩾20.0	–	–	4	2
TOTAL	12	14	12	12
Diastolic				
<5	10	7	3	2
5.0–9.9	2	7	3	2
10.0–14.9	–	–	6	8
15.0–19.9	–	–	–	–
⩾20.0	–	–	–	–
TOTAL	12	14	12	12

[a]For each age–sex group, the mean blood pressure of whites was subtracted from that of the corresponding Negro group. This difference was classified as to magnitude and counted in that group.
Source: Borhani and Borkham.[23]

comparison of age–sex groups by size of difference (between races) reveals that two thirds of the Alameda and nearly one half of the National Health Survey groups have less than 5 mmHg difference between the mean blood pressure of corresponding white and black persons.[23,39] In contrast, the Muscogee and Evans County[18] studies show only one fifth of their age–sex groups revealing this low interracial difference, while about one third were in the range of 15 mmHg or more difference.

The suggestion that real and significant intraracial variation in blood pressure does in fact exist in this country is supported by observed intraracial variation documented in other parts of the world. Epstein and Eckoff's[41] tabulation of racial–regional differences in mean blood pressure from many populations across the world (in terms of absolute level and slope of mean curve with age) displays many examples of intraracial variation. Lovell[42] also undertook a review of critical literature on intraracial variation in blood pressure. He concludes that differences between races are not great compared to the considerable variation within races. Perhaps even more dramatic than these intraracial differences observed between studies are the significant intraracial differences within two carefully conducted large-scale studies.[20, 22] In the blood pressure survey of the total adult population of Bergen, Norway, systematic and significant differences in the distribution and mean levels of pressure are observed between two geographic areas; housing condition is the only environmental factor to which such variation can be attributed.[22] Miall and Lovell[20] hypothesize that seasonal variation in pressure is most likely responsible for the systematic variation in pressure observed between the two populations in South Wales.

Examination of the intraracial differences displayed in the five United States studies of biracial populations—the three southern studies, on the one hand, and the nationwide and the California samples, on the other—thus suggests that this variation could be due to environmental factors associated with region. Yet, when the nationwide data is analyzed to determine if significant variation in blood pressure by race is found between areas of the country (the South, in particular), only minor differences are revealed. A further analysis[39] was undertaken to determine whether the interracial difference in mean pressure was significant. It was hypothesized that an interracial mean difference of the magnitude observed (about 5 mmHg) could be entirely caused by differential stress in the examination situation. The difference between the first and third casual measurements for the races was thus calculated. It was hypothesized that if tension was a significant determinant of blood pressure variation in Negroes, pressure would show a greater drop between the first and the third readings. This is in fact the case, and the conclusion is reached that at least "part of the recorded racial difference in blood pressure readings may arise from greater tension on the part of the Negro examinee at the time of the examination." However, this explanation does not account for the interracial differences in the prevalence rates of enlarged left ventricles, electrocardiographic abnormalities, or increased mortality from hypertension, all of which are higher in blacks than whites. Large interracial differences in blood pressure commonly attributed to biologic difference might, in fact, be due primarily to environmental factors. Most investigators agree that racial variation in blood pressure needs to be carefully considered not only with respect to age and sex, but also in the context of socioeconomic (occupation),[18, 23, 37, 43] sociocultural (stress),[25, 29, 33, 37, 42] dietary (salt intake),[7, 18, 35, 45] and biomedical (body build)[18, 33, 42, 45, 46] variables. These environmental factors are dealt with below.

SOCIOECONOMIC FACTORS

Occupation Of all related socioeconomic variables occupation is perhaps the most difficult to assess in terms of its effect on blood pressure. This is due in large measure to the confusion in the literature as to what is the relevant dimension of "occupation"—a measure of activity status, psychological stress, prestige, or a combination of these. An attempt has been made below to present the findings in terms of activity and stress, although it is recognized that it is often difficult to objectively rate occupations by these dimensions.

Activity Status It is a long-standing finding that strenuous physical exercise has immediate cardiovascular consequences in most individuals.[47] The relationship between habitual activity status (usually measured by use of an occupational index) and blood pressure is less clear.[47]

Conflicting evidence comes from major European studies. Lowe's[21] well-known study of the physical demands of occupation in relation to blood pressure, conducted on a large, British, employed population produces the following observations: no significant trend in women, no significant trend in men under 40 years of age, significantly higher mean systolic pressures in men engaged in more physically strenuous occupations.

Using age-adjusted scores, Miall[7] demonstrates that men 50 years or older, engaged in heavy labor most of their lives, have significantly lower blood pressures than other groups. Moreover, those in the least physically demanding occupations have the highest pressures, and the intermediate group the intermediate pressures. A 4-year follow-up of the same population revealed a similar pattern. Significantly, younger males with less occupational experience do not exhibit this association.

An association between blood pressure and activity status is sought in the Framingham data using two measures: physical activity index* and direct hand grip (dynamometer). No relationship can be established between blood pressure and either of these measures in the "relatively sedentary" Framingham population. Similarly, findings from the National Health Examination[43] on the relation between

---

*Calculated on the basis of the usual hours per day reported spent sleeping, sedentary awake, walking, and moderate and strenuous activity; multiplied by the appropriate figure for the associated increase in O_2 consumption.

prevalence of hypertension and usual activity status are not definitive. The evidence for the association of activity status and blood pressure remains unconvincing.[23, 47, 48] The confusion in the literature might be explained in terms of failure to control for body build factors, length of employment, socioeconomic status, or selective mortality. In general, the findings support the conclusion of Henry and Cassel[48] that variations in amount of habitual physical exercise are insufficient to explain variation in blood pressure observed in most populations. In a comprehensive review of worldwide literature on this association, they find support for each of the following contradictory associations: high blood pressure and high exercise, high blood pressure and low exercise, low blood pressure and high exercise, and low blood pressure and low exercise.

Occupation-Related Stress Information on this dimension of occupation is similarly fragmentary and inconsistent. Several Russian studies have implicated mental strain as an etiologic factor in the genesis of elevated pressure and report the therapeutic value of a change in jobs for such cases.[1, 49] Findings of Morrison and Morris[50] on a population of London bus drivers and conductors point in the same direction; the more mentally taxing job of driver is associated with higher pressures. In contrast, Lowe's[21] working population reveals a tendency for systolic pressures in men over 40 to increase with decreasing mental demands of occupation. Similarly, in Bergen, Humerfelt and Wedervang[51] find that the lowest prevalences of elevated pressures are associated with professions and those in more responsible occupational positions exhibited lower mean pressures than those in more subordinate positions.

No solid evidence in support of this association is found in the United States studies. Findings on the prevalence of elevated pressures from the National Health Survey[43] in relation to this occupational stress factor are difficult to interpret because of the nature of the occupational classification employed. However, a significant finding is a lower-than-expected prevalence among professionals in both races in each sex. Similarly, while few differences are observed among currently working males, Negroes of the Alameda sample[23] in "white collar" jobs were not proportionately represented in the upper quartile of systolic values.

Findings from studies on the influence of occupation on blood pressure produce no clear trend and are particularly confusing in light of the association of two occupation dimensions examined here (that is, mentally stressful occupations tend to be sedentary, and vice versa). Often, studies fail to control for length of employment; rarely do they mention work conditions; sometimes they do not take into account the relevant influence of body build factors. The complex relationships between occupation and blood pressure are reviewed by Howard and Holman.[52] At present it is impossible to estimate the influence of occupation on blood pressure.

Education   Three large-scale U.S. studies[23, 43, 47] report a significant association between educational status and blood pressure. In the nationwide probability sample,[43] prevalence of hypertensive pressures (160 and/or 95+ mmHg) was shown to be associated with education in both races. Among whites, there appears to be a steady trend toward a lower prevalence for those with greater education; in Caucasians and Negroes with less than 5 years of education, prevalence rates of definite hypertension were higher than expected (Table 4). Findings from the Alameda biracial sample[23] relating mean blood pressure to education reveal a similar pattern.

Cross-sectional analysis of the Framingham data[47] does not reveal a significant effect of educational status on blood pressure distributions. However, the mean systolic blood pressure of the most highly educated group in each decade of both sexes is found to be lower than in less-educated groups, with statistically significant differences appearing in

TABLE 4   Actual and Expected Prevalence Rates (Percent) of Definite Hypertension in Adults, by Race, Education, and Sex in the United States, 1960–1962

Years of Education	Men			Women		
	Actual	Expected	Difference	Actual	Expected	Difference
White						
Under 5	26.9	19.6	7.3	36.5	28.2	8.3
5–8	16.1	16.9	−0.7	26.4	23.0	3.4
9–12	10.7	10.5	0.1	10.3	11.4	−1.1
13 and over	9.3	10.3	−0.9	9.5	12.7	−3.3
Negro						
Under 5	42.9	37.7	5.2	46.3	41.4	4.9
5–8	27.8	29.9	−2.1	33.3	34.3	−1.0
9–12	18.3	18.4	−0.1	17.1	17.1	0.0
13 and over	15.5	22.5	−7.0	14.9	20.2	−5.3

Source: National Center for Health Statistics.[43]

the two upper decades.[34-46, 53-59] This finding is noteworthy in a population as relatively homogeneous as the Framingham sample.

Income and Other Socioeconomic Indices Analysis of the National Health Examination[43] data includes an assessment of prevalence of pressures 160 and/or 95+ mmHg by family income. No pattern of prevalence is found associated with family income in whites. In blacks with incomes below $7,000 per year, clear differentials in prevalence are observed, "with higher than expected prevalences both for men and women with family incomes of less than $2,000. . ."[43] (Table 5). Significantly, this race–income finding is found to be modified by area of residence (Table 6).

In the Alameda study[23] mean blood pressure is analyzed by family income in race–sex–age groups. Similar to the National Health Survey findings, family income is not consistently associated with pressure in whites, and correlation coefficients for systolic blood pressure and income are low. Significant differences are noted among the following Negro groups: Males under 45 and females over 45 with low family incomes (less than $4,000) have higher mean systolic blood pressure than middle- or high-income groups; males over 45 with high family

TABLE 5 Actual and Expected Prevalence Rates (Percent) of Definite Hypertension in Adults, by Race, Family Income, and Sex in the United States, 1960–1962

Family Income	Men			Women		
	Actual	Expected	Difference	Actual	Expected	Difference
White						
Under $2,000	16.7	18.3	−1.6	30.3	25.5	4.9
$2,000–3,999	13.9	13.5	0.4	16.3	17.0	−0.7
$4,000–6,999	12.2	11.2	1.0	10.3	11.5	−1.2
$7,000–9,999	10.6	11.1	−0.5	11.5	12.1	−0.7
$10,000 or over	11.6	13.2	−1.6	11.9	13.5	−1.6
Unknown	14.6	13.2	1.4	20.1	18.4	1.7
Negro						
Under $2,000	37.1	29.8	7.3	34.8	30.5	4.3
$2,000–3,999	21.6	26.9	−5.4	24.7	22.9	1.9
$4,000–6,999	20.3	23.7	−3.4	19.1	25.0	−6.0
$7,000–9,999	5.4	19.2	−13.8	22.1	22.5	−0.4
$10,000 or over	26.6	20.0	6.5	—	5.6	−5.6
Unknown	35.3	28.3	7.0	16.6	28.0	−11.4

Source: National Center for Health Statistics.[43]

TABLE 6   Race Differentials in Prevalence of Definite Hypertension (160 and/
or 95+ mmHg) among Persons with Family Incomes of Less Than $2,000, by
Place of Residence

Geographic Location	White	Negro
Metropolitan areas		
Men	11.6	13.7
Women	8.3	21.8
Rural South		
Men	15.4	31.5
Women	19.5	36.7

Source: National Center for Health Statistics.[43]

income ($8,000–9,999) have higher mean diastolic pressures than the
low-income group. No explanation is offered for the inconsistency of
the observed relation between blood pressure and family income in
older versus younger Negro men.

Remarkably, although many investigators have hypothesized socioeconomic status to be a significant determinant of observed blood
pressure variation, little work has been done in this area to date. The
most significant findings from U.S. studies in this connection come
from the Alameda survey.[23] An index of socioeconomic status
(based on averaging education, occupation, and income levels) is
found to be inversely related to blood pressure in both races. Differences observed are larger among Negroes than among Caucasians. Differences are larger in the 35–54-year age group than in either youngest
or oldest groups. It is of interest that the mean systolic pressure is
similar for middle-class blacks and whites. A parallel trend is observed
in correlation coefficients for mean systolic blood pressure and socioeconomic status, with significant negative associations appearing in
the following groups: white males age 35–44; white females age 45–54;
and Negro males under 45.

The literature on social class and blood pressure has many weaknesses. Interpretation of the existing data is made even more difficult
because of the interrelationships of the various socioeconomic factors
and their association with many possible etiologic agents, e.g., diet
and—perhaps most important—health care utilization. Thus, it is important to control for the use of antihypertensive drugs. One might
expect the greater utilization of medical care to be at least partially
reflected in the generally documented trend for blood pressures to be

inversely related to socioeconomic factors, but conclusions on the relevance of this variable remain tenuous.

BODY BUILD

Many investigators have postulated that, in addition to age, body build is the other most important determinant of blood pressure. This association is suggested by clinical experience[54] indicating that many hypertensives were obese and that weight reduction was often an effective therapeutic procedure. Subsequently, both cross-sectional and longitudinal surveys[1, 33, 54, 56] have consistently demonstrated a direct relationship between measures of body build/bulk and blood pressure levels. This relationship is generally most evident in young and middle-aged adults,[33, 56] whites,[19, 23, 28] and women.[22, 28, 55]

The National Health Examination data[28] include a comprehensive analysis of this variable in relation to blood pressure in the nationwide sample. Relevant measures taken at the time of the standardized examination included standing height, weight (partly dressed), right triceps and infrascapular skinfold, and arm girth. A weak inverse correlation is found between mean blood pressure and height, while the correlation coefficients for systolic and diastolic pressure for all race-sex groups and weight are direct and significant.

In the Alameda study[23] measures of body build are also found to be most significantly related to blood pressure in whites. The results of this study can be summarized as follows: For systolic pressure, weight indices and blood pressure are significantly correlated in white males and females 55 years of age or less, and in Negro females 45 years or less; significant diastolic correlations are found for white males of all ages and white females 45 years or less. No significant correlations are found in either diastolic or systolic pressure for Negroes 45 years of age or more.

Several other cross-sectional studies of large representative white populations in Europe and the United States have investigated the relationship of body build measures to blood pressure. In his analysis of the South Wales data, Lovell[42] finds the expected association between mean pressures within age groups and direct weight, with heavier individuals tending to have higher mean pressures. Similar to the National Health Examination findings,[28] this relationship is more marked in females for both systolic and diastolic.

In the first longitudinal study to investigate the association between body build and blood pressure, Harlan[32] demonstrates significant positive associations in a population of healthy males followed-up 18 years after their initial examination. Simple correlations calculated from the 1940 and 1958 examinations reveal that various measures of body build exerted insignificant influence on blood pressure in the young, healthy population, but 18 years later several measures of body build show significant positive association with blood pressure.

An employed male cohort was also investigated longitudinally by Stamler[58] with respect to weight and blood pressure trends over 20 years of observation. When the prevalence of final diastolic pressures 90 mmHg or more and 95 mmHg or more are analyzed by first relative weight (first actual weight divided by desirable weight calculated from standard life insurance tables for height) and slope of weight gain over the 20-year interval, a striking positive association is demonstrated between prevalence of elevated levels and weight gain and between prevalence and weight gain relative to initial relative weight (Figure 8).

Investigators analyzing longitudinal data from the Framingham cohort[54] find a straightforward association between weight gain and change in pressure over 12 years of observation. Those individuals who gain weight over the period of observation experience a substantial increase in systolic pressure, while pressures dropped in those losing weight. Significantly, when change in systolic pressure is analyzed by change in relative weight, the positive association is more marked in males; this is in contrast to most reports documenting a closer association between body build variables and blood pressure in women. Analysis of risk of developing hypertensive blood pressure levels (160 and/or 95+ mmHg) by weight change reveals increased risk rising proportionately with weight gain. Risk of developing hypertensive levels over 12 years is also shown to be significantly associated with relative weight on initial exam, mean relative weight over the entire period of observation, and relative weight at each biennial exam. Moreover, individuals with initial pressure levels less than 160/95 who are also in the highest relative weight groups show an excess risk of developing hypertensive levels relative to those with initially lower relative weights.

Many problems emerge in the interpretation of data on body build. Several investigators question the reliability and sensitivity of such measurements.[33, 35, 54, 60] Despite the high intercorrelation of body build variables and blood pressure, there remains confusion as to which factor, e.g., relative weight, body bulk, adiposity, and type of obesity, is actually associated with elevated blood pressure in any

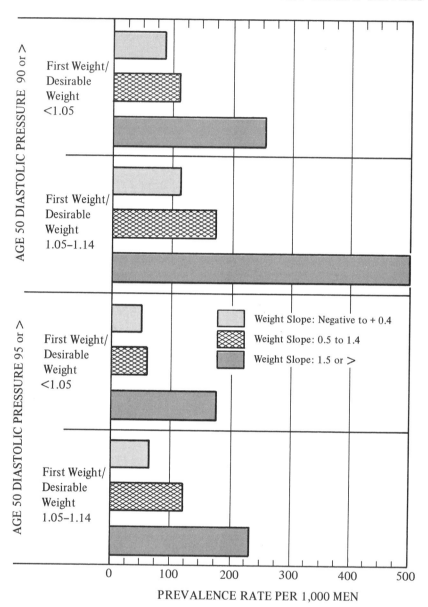

FIGURE 8 Twenty-year follow-up data on 746 men, age 40–59: young adult first weight, 20-year weight slope, and development of hypertensive disease in middle age. Reprinted by permission from Stamler J: Discussion of body composition and elevated blood pressure, The Epidemiology of Hypertension. Edited by J Stamler, R Stamler, TN Pullman, New York, Grune & Stratton, Inc, p 105, 1967.

given population.[54, 58, 59, 61] Indeed, some investigators contend that the correlation of body build measures and blood pressure might be the result of the association of these two factors with a third, e.g., socioeconomic status,[62] diet,[2] or age.[22]

Regardless of the genesis of the relationship, general findings reported in longitudinal and cross-sectional studies reviewed above support the significant direct association of weight-related factors and increases in blood pressure. This trend is more marked in whites, in females, and in young and middle-aged adults. In combination with age, measures of body build appear to account for a large proportion of the variance in blood pressure observed in Western populations.

DIETARY AND RELATED FACTORS

Despite the weaknesses inherent in dietary studies, many investigators believe that dietary factors are associated with blood pressure variation.[47] Kempner,[63] the originator of the therapeutic rice–fruit diet, was one of the first to suggest this association. He believes that the benefit of his dietary regimen is due to its low animal protein content; its effectiveness is attributed by others to its low sodium content.

Sodium   Sodium chloride was originally implicated as a factor associated with blood pressure variation on the basis of therapeutic success of low sodium diets in reducing pressure in hypertensives.[64] Dahl[65] and Meneely *et al.*[66] undertook extensive animal investigations of the relationship between sodium intake and hypertension. These studies demonstrate that experimental hypertension, with accompanying target organ complications and mortality, can be induced in rats by a high sodium diet; not all strains of rats are equally susceptible to the hypertensive effects of increased salt intake. In susceptible strains the degree of morbidity is parallel to the level of salt intake.

Dahl and Love[67] find a significant association between mean blood pressures of 1,300 American male employees (age 20–69) at Brookhaven Laboratories taken during routine physical exams and general level of salt intake throughout life (judged by amount of salt added at the table). Those judged on low salt intake experience a lower prevalence of elevated pressure levels. Two studies of Japanese populations find measurement of 24-hour urinary chloride and sodium excretions to be correlated with the prevalence of elevated blood pressure.[64] Dahl, cited by Evans and Rose,[33] studied the relationship between mean blood pressure and salt intake as measured by urinary sodium output from studies on various populations. His results demonstrate a significant positive correlation between prevalence of elevated pressure and measures of salt intake. However, data from other studies[1, 12, 33, 47, 48] have failed to document such an association. In a cross-sectional analysis of the Framingham data[47] no relation is demonstrated when salt intake is estimated from dietary interview, 24-hour urine output, or sodium potassium-to-urine ratio.

Despite these conflicting reports, many investigators[12, 47] believe that sodium intake is a significant environmental factor related to blood pressure variation. The lack of association documented in some studies may be attributed to problems in the accurate estimation of sodium intake, to the failure to control for other variables that might influence this association (e.g., weight), or simply the possibility that sodium intake may not affect the blood pressure of all populations.

In addition to sodium intake, other dietary factors have been implicated. Some general statements can be made about these factors in specific populations whose diet varies little with respect to certain nutritional components. Intake of animal or vegetable fat does not appear associated with blood pressure level. The milk-drinking Samburu nomads of Kenya[68] and other populations with high-protein, high-fat diets[48] have low mean blood pressures, exhibit no significant rise in pressure with age, and have a very low prevalence of elevated pressures despite their high-fat diets. Conversely, in certain populations with extremely low fat intake, such as urban Japanese[69] and Uganda villagers,[45] elevated pressure is not uncommon. One carefully conducted study of two complete Japanese villages with contrasting cardiovascular mortality rates[70] finds that residents of the villages do not differ in height, weight, serum lipid values, or salt intake (high sodium intake in both). Significant differences are found, however, in mean blood pressure of both sexes and in the intake of certain vitamins and minerals, especially vitamin A, riboflavin, and ascorbic acid. The authors hypothesize that high salt intake in combination with low intake of some vitamins predisposes toward elevated blood pressure. However, the Framingham dietary evaluation[47] fails to reveal an association when systolic pressure quartiles for age–sex groups were investigated in relation to mean daily intake of calories, protein, fat, and cholesterol and in simple correlation analysis.

Other Factors   Among the short-term cardiovascular effects known to be associated with smoking are increases in pulse, cardiac output, and peripheral resistance, as well as change in ECG patterns.[47] Systolic pressure increases of 5–35 mmHg have been recorded, although in some individuals no increase is apparent; diastolic pressure varies only slightly.[47] Most investigations of the effect of cigarette smoking on blood pressure variation show no clear trend or slightly lower mean pressures in smokers.[7, 23, 33, 47, 71] In addition, many investigators suggest that when an inverse relationship is found, it is likely to be a reflection of body weight differences with smokers tending to weigh less.[11, 33, 71]

Similarly, the association of blood pressure variation with trace metal concentrations and the hardness of drinking water remains unclear. The latter data rest solely on mortality statistics.[47, 72] Further clinical investigation is needed to directly implicate trace metals as a significant factor in blood pressure variation.

In a study[28] on the relationship between systolic and diastolic blood pressure and age, body measurements, blood glucose, and serum glucose, correlations and multiple regression analyses were carried out. Blood glucose is found to be significantly correlated with both systolic and diastolic blood pressure after the effects of age, physique, and race are removed. When similar multiple regression analyses are performed with serum cholesterol, the correlation between blood pressure and cholesterol is found only with blood pressure and white men, and even this is minimal. The authors conclude that "the simple correlation found between cholesterol and blood pressure must be indirect, and due to the correlation of each with physique—especially bulk—and age."[28]

FAMILIAL AGGREGATION

Many physicians have the clinical impression that high blood pressure "runs in families."[1, 35, 56, 73, 74] The increased prevalence of hypertension has been documented in siblings and offspring of hypertensives in comparison to controls[32, 56, 75, 76] Studies of twins report concordance in pressure between monozygotic twins[35, 75] and large scale epidemiologic studies[14, 44, 76] yield statistical evidence quantifying the trend toward familial aggregation at all levels of blood pressure. Miall *et al.* evaluated family aggregation of pressures in his South Wales[27] and Jamaica[44] populations. The most striking finding is that the resemblance in pressure between close relatives is independent of the range of pressure considered, an observation documented earlier by Hamilton *et al.*[26] Results from the Tecumseh, Michigan study[14, 76] are essentially in agreement with those of Hamilton and Miall.

In combination with the trends in blood pressure by race, these findings on familial aggregation suggest that genetic factors may play a role in blood pressure variation. The relative contribution of genetic and environmental factors is always difficult to evaluate. However, Pickering[3] points out that the correlation coefficients (r) found in the previously quoted studies of family aggregation are quite low, approximately 0.2, in comparison to the correlation coefficients expected if blood pressure variation were controlled by a dominant gene (approximately 0.5). It has been suggested that environmental factors alone could be responsible for family aggregation of blood pressure, due to the tendency of related persons to share the same or very similar environments;[7, 41, 77] this argument would appear to find support in the documented blood pressure changes of persons migrating to a new environment.[3] Some studies[14, 76, 78] of familial aggregation attempt to control for environmental factors by comparing blood pressures of relatives and those of spouses. There is no significant correlation between spouses' pressures, and their correlation coefficients are significantly different from those found between relatives; these findings are not altered when the period of time the spouses had lived together is controlled.[14] It thus appears that genetic factors do play a role in determining variation in pressure, although, as Pickering suggests,[3] it might be limited to an influence on initial pressure level and independent of subsequent rate of rise.

PSYCHOLOGICAL AND SOCIOCULTURAL FACTORS

Psychological and sociocultural factors are presumed by many to be responsible for a significant portion of blood pressure variation. The evidence in support of this association is fragmentary, due, in no small measure, to the inherent difficulties in defining and measuring these variables.

The focus of much early work on psychological factors is on the definition of the "hypertensive personality."[10, 79-81] An apparent weakness of this type of study is the inability to determine whether the personality syndrome gives rise to the elevated pressure or whether it is an outcome of the elevated pressure.[41, 79] Wolf et al.'s[82] extensive investigation of pressor responses in hyper- and normotensive individuals to psychological stress establishes that acutely stressful occurrences, whether of objective or subjective origin, can induce transient elevations of blood pressure in some individuals. It is still not established, however, whether repetition of, or continuous, psychological stress results in sustained pressure elevation.[1, 10, 33, 80, 83]

In a cross-sectional investigation of a large male employed population (age 40–55), Ostfeld and Shekelle[80] relate objective psychological test scores (MMPI, Catell 16 Personal Factor) to blood pressure. Pressures are identified that are one standard deviation or more above or below the group mean, and pairs of highs and lows are matched for age and arm girth. No significant relationship can be established between any personality factor and these extreme blood pressure groups.

A classic study of sociocultural variables is the work of Scotch *et al.* among the Zulus in South Africa.[84, 85] Systematic random samples were taken of an urban relocation project in Durban and a rural native reserve nearby. Standardized blood pressure measurements and interviews were conducted. A pilot study had previously identified an increased prevalence of elevated diastolic (90+ mmHg) and higher mean pressures among the newly urbanized group. These differences were apparently not attributable to race, climate, age, diet, or selective migration to the city. A stress factor involved in sociocultural transition was thus hypothesized and an interview designed to elicit information on potential stress factors. When significant correlates of prevalence of elevated diastolic pressure (90+ mmHg) are analyzed for the two communities, the following are observed: (a) whether or not a particular element was stressful depends on its social context; and (b) in the urban community the variables related to prevalence of hypertension show a definite pattern, indicating that the individuals most likely to be hypertensive maintain traditional cultural practices incongruent with their new surroundings.

In this country some related work has been done in recent years. On the basis of a small pilot study of Negro males (age 30–49) residing in the Chicago slums (most of whom had recently migrated from the rural South), Stamler *et al.*[36] conclude that psychosocial factors reflecting stress versus adaptation to surroundings may be relevant to the distribution of elevated pressures within this racially homogeneous urban population. A more extensive study of similar variables within an urban community is being conducted in Detroit[86, 87] Carefully selected samples were chosen from two high-stress and two low-stress neighborhoods (based on socioeconomic level, crime rate, overcrowding, etc.). Each stress category included one predominantly black and one predominantly white population. Preliminary analyses reveal significantly higher prevalence (2:1) of pressures 160 and/or 95+ mmHg in the high-stress neighborhoods versus low-stress neighborhoods of the same race. These results could not be attributed to age, sex, or weight differences.

Review of the literature on psychological and sociocultural variables in the distribution of blood pressure reveals that most studies suffer from serious weaknesses in sampling and controls.[79] However, recent investigations have employed increasingly sophisticated measures of sociological variables such as mobility and incongruity in relation to blood pressure. While work in this area is in its infancy, it is a potentially fruitful direction for future research.

It is generally agreed that there is a need to apply sociological theory in the formulation of future hypotheses concerning these psychological and sociocultural relationships. Furthermore, it would be useful to develop such theoretical concepts into operational instruments that could be used in future epidemiological studies.[23, 25, 36, 76, 81, 88-90]

FUNCTIONAL IMPACT

Longitudinal studies of patients with essential hypertension reveal that most cases develop between age 35 and 45.[91] A sudden rise in blood pressure prior to age 30 or after age 50 might indicate secondary hypertension caused by adrenal, renal, or specific vascular lesions. It is not unusual to find in long-term follow-up studies of essential hypertension that blood pressure in approximately 50 percent of patients remains unchanged from 5 to 10 years. Indeed, Bechgaard[92] finds in a study of 1,038 patients with essential hypertension that of those who survived to the second examination, 61 percent maintained the same blood pressure, 12 percent recorded an increase, and 27 percent a decrease.

Although essential hypertension is often associated with headaches, vertigo, dyspnea on exertion, nosebleeds, nervousness, and chest pain, the frequency of these symptoms and the relationship to hypertension has not been carefully defined. Many of these symptoms are common in the general adult population and may be attributed erroneously to a patient's hypertension. Long-term follow-up studies, however, do reveal that 50 to 80 percent[92] of patients with hypertension will develop cardiac enlargement. The common causes of death with hypertension[93] are coronary heart disease, cerebral vascular disease, and renal failure.

In a study by the Society of Actuaries[94] of five million insured persons, 200,000 are found to have had a casual blood pressure between 140 and 170 mmHg systolic and between 90 and 115 mmHg diastolic on their life insurance examination. For the most part these insured persons are free of other known conditions, except obesity. Analysis of this sample of persons with essential hypertension but without serious complications documents the effect of mild hypertension on mortality. Men with a casual blood pressure 140 mmHg systolic and 90 mmHg diastolic are subject to about a 50 percent increase in mortality over 20 years, compared with the average of all insured lives. This risk increases to 100 percent when the blood pressure is 145/95 and to 200 percent when the pressure is 160/100.

There is ample data to verify that chemotherapy of malignant hypertension improves the patient's prognosis.[95] Treatment of this severe type of hypertension reduces deaths from cerebral vascular disease and renal failure but does not affect the death rate from myocardial infarction.[95] Although there is controversy over the impact of treatment of borderline essential hypertension (diastolic pressure 90–104 mmHg), the Veterans Administration Cooperative Study indicates clearly that patients with moderate hypertension (diastolic pressure 115–129 mmHg) respond to therapy.[96, 97] For the most part, the beneficial effects are due to a reduction in cardiovascular episodes; however, as is the case with treatment of malignant hypertension, the incidence of myocardial infarction remains unchanged.[98] In a recent review of the effects of antihypertensive therapy, Freis[99] documents reduced morbidity and mortality in male hypertensives, with a mean diastolic pressure as low as 105 mmHg regardless of age.

REFERENCES

1. Schweitzer MD, Gearing FR, Perara GA: The epidemiology of primary hypertension. Present status. J Chron Dis 18:847–857, 1965
2. Rasmussen P: An overview of essential hypertension. Med Times 95: 467–476, 1967
3. Pickering G: Hypertension: Causes, Consequences and Management. London, J & A Churchill, 1970
4. Enigma of hypertension. Br Med J 5469:1011–1012, 1965
5. Stamler J, Stamler R, Pullman TN: The Epidemiology of Hypertension. New York, Grune & Stratton, Inc, 1967
6. National Center for Health Statistics: Blood Pressure of Adults by Age and Sex, United States, 1960–1962. Department of Health, Education, and Welfare, Washington, DC, Government Printing Office, 1964. (Vital and Health Statistics Series 11, No 4)
7. Miall WE: The epidemiology of essential hypertension, Proceedings: Symposium on Pathogenesis of Essential Hypertension. Edited by JH Cort, V Fencl, Z Hejl, J Jirka. Oxford, Pergamon Press, 1962, pp 88–102
8. Fries ED: Discussion of the epidemiology of essential hypertension, Proceed-

ings: Symposium on Pathogenesis of Essential Hypertension. Edited by JH Cort, V Fencl, Z Hejl, J Jirka. Oxford, Pergamon Press, 1962, pp 103–125

9. Ostfeld AM, Lebovitz BZ: Blood pressure lability: A correlative study. J Chron Dis 12:428–439, 1960

10. McKegney FP, Williams RB, Jr: Psychological aspects of hypertension. II. The differential influence of interview variables on blood pressure. Am J Psych 123:1539–1545, 1967

11. Epstein FH: Epidemiologic studies on the nature of high blood pressure, Renal Metabolism and Epidemiology of Some Renal Diseases. Edited by J Metcoff. New York, National Kidney Foundation, 1964, pp 263–276

12. Maddocks I: Dietary factors in the genesis of hypertension, Proceedings of the Sixth International Congress on Nutrition. Edinburgh, Livingston Ltd, 1963

13. Feinleib M, Gordon T, Kannel WB, Garrison RJ: Relationship between blood pressure and age. The Framingham study. Paper presented at the Tenth Annual Conference on Cardiovascular Disease Epidemiology, New Orleans, March 2 and 3, 1970

14. Johnson BC, Epstein FH, Kjelsberg MO: Distributions and familial studies of blood pressure and serum cholesterol levels in a total community—Tecumseh, Mich. J Chron Dis 18:147–160, 1965

15. Kagan A, Gordon T, Kannel WB, et al: Blood pressure and its relation to coronary heart disease in the Framingham Study. Hypertension, Vol VII. Chicago, American Heart Association, 1959, pp 53–81

16. Comstock GW: An epidemiologic study of blood pressure levels in a biracial community in the southern US Am J Hyg 65:271–315, 1957

17. Johnson BC, Remington RD: A sampling study of blood pressure levels in white and Negro residents of Nassau, Bahamas. J Chron Dis 13:39–51, 1969

18. McDonough JR, Garrison GE, James CG: Blood pressure and hypertensive disease among Negroes and whites in Evans County, Georgia, The Epidemiology of Hypertension. Edited by J Stamler, R Stamler, T N Pullman. New York, Grune & Stratton, Inc, 1967, pp 167–187

19. Boyle W, Griffey WP, Nichaman MZ, et al: An epidemiologic study of hypertension among racial groups of Charleston County, South Carolina. The Charleston heart study, Phase II, The Epidemiology of Hypertension. Edited by J Stamler, R Stamler, TN Pullman. New York, Grune & Stratton, Inc. 1967, pp 193–203

20. Miall WE, Lovell HG: Relation between change of blood pressure and age. Br Med J 2:660–664, 1967

21. Lowe CR: Arterial pressure, physique and occupation. Br J Prev Soc Med 18:115–125, 1964

22. Boe J, Humerfelt S, Wedervang F: The blood pressure in a population. Acta Med Scand 157 (Suppl 321):1–336, 1957

23. Borhani NO, Borkman TS: The Alameda County blood pressure study. Berkeley, State of California Department of Public Health, 1968

24. Ueda S, Yano K: ABCC-JNIH Adult Health Study, Hiroshima 1958–60. Hiroshima-Nagasaki, Japan. Atomic Bomb Casualty Commission, Japanese National Institute of Health, 1962

25. Lin TY, Hung TP, Chen CM, et al: A study of normal and elevated blood

pressure in a Chinese urban population in Taiwan. Clin Sci 18:301–312, 1959

26. Hamilton M, Pickering GW, Fraser-Roberts JA, et al: The etiology of essential hypertension. I. The arterial pressure in the general population. Clin Sci 13:11–35, 1954

27. Miall WE, Oldham PK: A study of arterial pressure and its inheritance in a sample of the general population. Clin Sci 14:459–488, 1955

28. Florey C duV, Acheson RM: Blood pressure as it relates to physique, blood glucose and serum cholesterol, US 1960–1962. Department of Health, Education, and Welfare, Washington, DC, Government Printing Office, 1969 (Vital and Health Statistics Series 11, No 34)

29. Florey C duV, Cuadrado RR: Blood pressure in native Cape Verdeans and in Cape Verdean immigrants and their descendants in New England. Hum Biol 40:189–211, 1968

30. Holland WW, Raftery EP, McPherson P, et al: A cardiovascular survey of American East Coast telephone workers. Am J Epidemiol 85:61–71, 1967

31. Stamler J, Lindberg HA, Berkson DM, et al: Prevalence and incidence of coronary heart disease in strata of the labor force of a Chicago industrial corporation. J Chron Dis 11:405–420, 1960

32. Harlan WR, Osborne RK, Graybiel A: A longitudinal study of blood pressure. Circulation 26:530–543, 1962

33. Evans JG, Rose G: Hypertension. Br Med Bull 27:37–42, 1971

34. Lukl P: Essential hypertension. WHO Chron 15:363–370, 1961

35. Geiger HJ, Scotch NA: The epidemiology of essential hypertension: A review with special attention to psychological and sociocultural factors. J Chron Dis 16:1151–1182, 1963

36. Stamler J, Berkson DM, Lindberg HA, et al: Socioeconomic factors in the epidemiology of hypertensive disease, The Epidemiology of Hypertension. Edited by J Stamler, R Stamler, TN Pullman. New York, Grune & Stratton, Inc, 1967, pp 289–313

37. Lennard HL, Block CY: Studies in hypertension: VI. Differences in the distribution of hypertension in Negroes and whites. An appraisal. J Chron Dis 5:186–196, 1957

38. Moser M: Epidemiology of hypertension with particular reference to racial susceptibility. Ann NY Acad Sci 18:989–999, 1960

39. National Center for Health Statistics: Blood pressure of adults by race and area, US 1960–1962. Department of Health, Education, and Welfare, Washington, DC, Government Printing Office, 1964 (Vital and Health Statistics Series 11, No 5)

40. Boyle E, Jr: Biological patterns in hypertension by race, sex, body weight and skin color. JAMA 213: 1637–1643, 1970

41. Epstein FH, Eckoff RD: The epidemiology of high blood pressure—geographic distributions and etiologic factors, The Epidemiology of Hypertension. Edited by J Stamler, R Stamler, TN Pullman. New York, Grune & Strattton, Inc, 1967, pp 155–166

42. Lovell RRH: Race and blood pressure, with special reference to Oceania, The Epidemiology of Hypertension. Edited by J Stamler, R Stamler, TN Pullman. New York, Grune & Stratton, Inc, 1967, pp 122–128

43. National Center for Health Statistics: Hypertension and hypertensive heart disease in adults, US 1960–1962. Department of Health, Education, and Welfare, Washington, DC, Government Printing Office, 1966 (Vital and Health Statistics Series 11, No 13)

44. Miall WE, Kass EH, Ling J, et al: Factors influencing arterial pressure in the general population in Jamaica. Br Med J 2:497–506, 1962

45. Shaper AG: Blood pressure studies in East Africa, The Epidemiology of Hypertension. Edited by J Stamler, R Stamler, TN Pullman. New York, Grune & Stratton, Inc, 1967, pp 139–145

46. Maddocks I: Blood pressure in Melanesians. Med J Aust 1:1123–1126, 1967

47. Dawber TR, Kannel WB, Kagan A, et al: Environmental factors in hypertension, The Epidemiology of Hypertension. Edited by J Stamler, R Stamler, TN Pullman. New York, Grune & Stratton, Inc, 1967, pp 255–282

48. Henry JP, Cassel JC: Psychological factors in essential hypertension: Recent epidemiologic and animal experimental evidence. Am J Epidemiol 90:171–200, 1969

49. Ryvkin IA, Maslova KK, Tiapina LA: The significance of employment and heredity in hypertensive disease. Cor Vasa 8:10–18, 1966

50. Morrison SL, Morris JN: Epidemiological observations on high blood pressure without evident cause. Lancet 2:864, 1959

51. Humerfelt S, Wedervang FR: A study of the influence upon blood pressure of marital status, number of children and occupation. Acta Med Scand 159:489–497, 1957

52. Howard J, Holman B: The effects of race and occupation on hypertension mortality. Milbank Mem Fund 48:263–296, 1970

53. Corcoran AC: Discussion of the epidemiology of essential hypertension, Proceedings: Symposium on Pathogenesis of Essential Hypertension. Edited by JH Cort, V Fencl, Z Hejl, J Jirka. Oxford, Pergamon Press, 1962, pp 103–125

54. Kannel WB, Brand N, Skinner JJ, et al: The relation of adiposity to blood pressure and development of hypertension: The Framingham Study. Ann Int Med 67:48–59, 1967

55. Miall WE, Bell RH, Lovell HG: Relation between change in blood pressure and weight. Br J Prev Soc Med 22:73–80, 1968

56. Moriyama IM, Stamler J, Krueger DE: Hypertensive disease, Cardiovascular Diseases of the United States. American Public Health Association. Harvard University Press, Cambridge, Massachusetts, 1971, pp 119–174 (Vital and Health Statistics Monographs)

57. Epstein FH, et al: Prevalence of chronic diseases and distribution of selected physiologic variables in a total community, Tecumseh, Michigan. Am J Epidemiol 81:307–322, 1965

58. Stamler J: Discussion of body composition and elevated blood pressure, The Epidemiology of Hypertension. Edited by J Stamler, R Stamler, TN Pullman. New York, Grune & Stratton, Inc, 1967, pp 104–109

59. Truedsson E: Variation of arterial blood pressure with age, sex, anthroposomatological dimensions, plasma lipids in the fasting state and after fat ingestion. Acta Med Scand (Suppl 381):1–76, 1962

60. Florey C duV: The use and interpretation of ponderal index and other weight–height ratios in epidemiologic studies. J Chron Dis 23:93–103, 1970

61. Ruzyllo E, Krotkiewski M, Kotowska A: Obesity and arterial hypertension. I. Hypertension in relation to the type of obesity. Bull Pol Med Sci Hist 10:54–57, 1967

62. Pell S, D'Alonzo CA: Chronic disease morbidity and income level in an employed population. Am J Public Health 60:116–129, 1970

63. Kempner W: Treatment of kidney disease and hypertensive vascular disease with rice diet. NC Med J 5:125–273, 1944

64. Moyer HJ: Hypertension: The 1st Hahnemann Symposium on Hypertensive Disease. Philadelphia, WB Saunders Co, 1959

65. Dahl LK: Effects of chronic excess salt ingestion—Experimental hypertension in the rat: Correlation with human hypertension, The Epidemiology of Hypertension. Edited by J Stamler, R Stamler, TN Pullman. New York, Grune & Stratton, Inc, 1967, pp 218–227

66. Meneely GR, Tucker RG, Darby WJ, et al: Chronic sodium chloride toxicity in albino rat. II. Occurrence of hypertension and of syndrome of edema and renal failure. J Exper Med 98:71, 1953

67. Dahl LK, Love RA: Etiological role of sodium chloride intake in essential hypertension in humans. JAMA 164:397, 1957

68. Shaper AG: Cardiovascular studies in the Samburu tribe of Northern Kenya. Am Heart J 63:437–442, 1962

69. Switzer S: Hypertension and Ischaemic heart disease in Hiroshima. Circulation 23:368–380, 1963

70. Kimura T, Ota M: Epidemiologic study of hypertension. Comparative results of hypertensive surveys in two areas in Northern Japan. Am J Clin Nutr 17:381–390, 1965

71. Ripka O, Srb V: Occurrence of arterial hypertension in Czechoslovakia. Rev Czech Med 11:149–160, 1965

72. Morton WE: Hypertension and drinking water constituents in Colorado. Paper presented at the epidemiology section, annual meeting of the APHA, Houston, Oct. 26–30, 1970

73. Inheritance of hypertension. Br Med J 5608:775–776, 1968

74. Schweitzer MD, Gearing FR, Perera GA: Family studies of primary hypertension: Their contribution to the understanding of genetic factors, The Epidemiology of Hypertension. Edited by J Stamler, R Stamler, TN Pullman. New York, Grune & Stratton, Inc, 1967, pp 28–37

75. Platt R: The influence of heredity, The Epidemiology of Hypertension. Edited by J Stamler, R Stamler, TN Pullman. New York, Grune & Stratton, Inc, 1967, pp 9–15

76. Deutscher S, Epstein FH, Kjelsberg MO: Familial aggregation of factors associated with coronary heart disease. Circulation 33:911–924, 1966

77. Trulson M: Subcommittee on methodology for diet appraisal. Am J Public Health 50 (Suppl 10):39–52, 1960

78. Miall WE, Moore F, Heanage P, et al: Blood pressure inheritance: An epidemiological study of populations in South Wales. Paper presented at the Epidemiological Council of the AHA, Chicago, 1966

79. Scotch NA, Geiger HJ: The epidemiology of essential hypertension: A review with special attention to psychological and sociocultural factors. J Chron Dis 16:1183–1213, 1963

80. Ostfeld AM, Shekelle RB: Psychological variables and blood pressure, The

Epidemiology of Hypertension. Edited by J Stamler, R Stamler, TN Pullman.
New York, Grune & Stratton, Inc, 1967, pp 321–331

81. Thomas CB: The psychological dimensions of hypertension, The Epidemiology of Hypertension. Edited by J Stamler, R Stamler, TN Pullman.
New York, Grune & Stratton, Inc, 1967, pp 332–339

82. Wolf S, Cardon PV, Jr, Shepard EM, et al: Life Stress and Essential Hypertension—A Study of Cardiovascular Adjustment in Man. Baltimore, Williams
& Wilkins, 1955

83. Shapiro AP: Psychophysiological aspects of blood pressure regulation:
Methodologic issues. Psychosom Med 26:481–509, 1964

84. Gampel B, Slome C, Scotch N, et al: Urbanization and hypertension among
Zulu adults. J Chron Dis 15:67–70, 1962

85. Scotch NA: Sociocultural factors in the epidemiology of Zulu hypertension.
Am J Public Health 53:1205–1213, 1963

86. Harburg E, Schull WJ, Erfurt JC, et al: A family set method for estimating
heredity and stress. I. J Chron Dis 23:69–81, 1970

87. Schull WJ, Harburg E, Erfurt JC, et al: A family set method for estimating
heredity and stress. II. J Chron Dis 23:83–92, 1970

88. Scotch NA: Discussion of psychological factors, The Epidemiology of Hypertension. Edited by J Stamler, R Stamler, TN Pullman. New York, Grune &
Stratton, Inc, 1967

89. Cruz-Coke R, Etcheverry R, Nagel R: Influence of migration on blood pressure of Easter Islanders. Lancet 1:697–699, 1964

90. Sive PH, Medalie JH, Kahn HA, et al: Distribution and multiple regression
analyses of blood pressure in 10,000 Israeli men. Am J Epidemiol
93:317–327, 1971

91. Perea GA: The natural history of hypertensive vascular disease, Hypertension,
A Symposium. Edited by ET Bell, University of Minnesota Press, 1950, p 363

92. Bechgaard P: The natural history of benign hypertension—One thousand
patients followed from 26 to 32 years, The Epidemiology of Hypertension.
Edited by J Stamler, R Stamler, TN Pullman. New York, Grune & Stratton,
Inc, 1967, pp 357–363,

93. Peart WS: Arterial hypertension, Cecil–Loeb Textbook of Medicine. Edited
by PB Berson, W McDermott, Philadelphia, WB Saunders Company, 1971,
p 1058

94. Lew EA: Blood pressure and mortality—Life insurance experience, The
Epidemiology of Hypertension. Edited by J Stamler, R Stamler, TN Pullman.
New York, Grune & Stratton, Inc, 1967, pp 392–397

95. Results of treatment of hypertension. Lancet 1:217–218, 1971

96. Veterans Administration: Cooperative Study Group on Antihypertensive
Agents: Effects of treatment on morbidity in hypertension. JAMA
202:1028–1034, 1967

97. Freis ED: Effectiveness of drug therapy in hypertension: Present status, a
review. Circ Res (suppl to vols XXVIII and XXIX), 1971

98. Veterans Administration Cooperative Study Group on Antihypertensive
Agents: Effects of treatment on morbidity in hypertension, II. Results in
patients with diastolic blood pressure averaging 90 through 114 mmHg.
JAMA 212:1143–1152, 1970

99. Freis ED: The treatment of hypertension why, when and how. Am J Med
52:664–671, 1972

BIBLIOGRAPHY

Report of Inter-Society Commission for Heart Disease Resources: Primary Prevention of Hypertension. Hypertension Study Group Circulation 42:A39–A41, 1970

Report of Inter-Society Commission for Heart Disease Resources: Resources for the Management of Emergencies in Hypertension. Hypertension Study Group Circulation 43:A157–A160, 1971

Report of Inter-Society Commission for Heart Disease Resources: Guidelines for the Detection, Diagnosis and Management of Hypertensive Populations. Hypertension Study Group Circulation 44:A263–A272, 1971

SIX

Urinary Tract Infections

SUMMARY

Which populations should be routinely screened for bacteriuria remains to be defined. However, the proper management of both asymptomatic and symptomatic urinary tract infections requires a careful history, selected physical examination, and a good understanding of the limitations of commonly used laboratory procedures. The provider of care must be able to interpret urinalyses and understand quantitative urine cultures. Because a variety of antimicrobial drugs, many with potentially serious side effects, is available for treatment, this tracer provides a discriminating tool for assessing the use of this common class of drugs. Appropriate follow-up and hospital use can be examined.

CLASSIFICATION

A clinical designation of urinary tract infection, bacteriuria, relies on the detection of a significant number of viable bacteria in the urine. The most widely accepted measure of significance is the quantitative colony count, established from observations by Kass and confirmed by many others. More than 100,000 organisms per ml of urine has come to be accepted as a reliable indication of the presence of a true infection.

162

EPIDEMIOLOGY

Age and Sex In general, the morbidity rates of bacteriuria increase with age for both males and females. Beginning in the preschool years and persisting for all subsequent ages until the geriatric years, the frequency of infection is significantly greater for females than males. It is reasonable to estimate that at least 5 percent of all girls will acquire bacteriuria at some point during the elementary and high school years, and that at least 10–20 percent of all adult women will experience an infection of the urinary tract in their lifetime. The pattern of increased frequency with age continues to persist for the geriatric age group, evidencing higher risk and greater severity of episodes than any other group. However, sex-related differences appear to diminish during these years.

Race The relationship of race to the distribution of bacteriuria has not been completely delineated. However, the consensus among investigators appears to be that race is not a major determinant of morbidity rates. The significance of higher rates among blacks observed by some researchers has been discounted by the intraracial differences documented among blacks and the similar rates between black and white groups of comparable social class.

Socioeconomic Status Although definitive epidemiologic studies are lacking, available data strongly indicate that socioeconomic status and morbidity rates are inversely related. Investigators have not determined whether this relationship reflects environmental factors or the availability and quality of medical care.

Pregnancy There is much data confirming a significant correlation between bacteriuria and pregnancy and documenting prevalence rates of 3–9 percent among pregnant women. The frequency of infection among pregnant women appears to be directly related to age and parity, but inversely related to the age at the time of first pregnancy. The cumulative effect of these variables has identified those pregnant women at particularly high risk who are of low socioeconomic status and either multiparous and over 30 years, or primiparous and under 20 years.

Other Factors Neither geographic location nor seasonal variation appears to be influential in the distribution of bacteriuria. Slight variations in rates have been reported by locality but can usually be explained on the basis of other variables. The seasonal variations in rate that have been documented appear to be correlated with the seasonal distribution of pregnancy.

Functional Impact   Long-term follow-up studies suggest that approximately 20–25 percent of women with bacteriuria spontaneously lose their infections annually and that a similar number become bacteriuric within the year. There are no reliable data on the distribution of urinary tract infections by site of infection, i.e., upper (kidney) versus lower (bladder) urinary tract. In addition to kidney infection, the other serious functional effects of urinary tract infection are the impact of asymptomatic bacteriuria on renal function and blood pressure and the relationship of bacteriuria during pregnancy to prematurity. In all of these associations, the data remain equivocal.

Kaitz, for example, has demonstrated a defect in ability to concentrate urine in a small group of women with asymptomatic bacteriuria. Several studies suggest that women with bacteriuria have a higher blood pressure than appropriate controls, and much confusion remains as to whether or not bacteriuric pregnant women are more likely to deliver premature babies. Kass *et al.,* also, have recently presented preliminary data suggesting that excess mortality exists among bacteriuric women. Despite the caveats that must be applied to these functional effects of urinary tract infections, these data indicate the potential significance of bacteriuria, although they do not define the magnitude of its impact.

A MINIMAL-CARE PLAN FOR SIGNIFICANT BACTERIURIA

I. Screening

A. *Quantitative urine culture.* (1) Pregnant women: once each trimester; (2) females: yearly, if history of previous urinary tract infections; (3) males and females with hypertension.

II. Evaluation (Initial Episode of Symptomatic or Asymptomatic Significant Bacteriuria)

A. *History.* (1) Presenting complaint; (2) previous bladder or kidney infection or kidney stone; (3) previous history of instrumentation or surgery (if yes, specify the date); (4) present history of dysuria, hematuria, frequency, nocturia; (5) pain [if yes, specify location: groin, lower abdomen, costovertebral angle (CVA), genitalia]; (6) fever, chills; (7) history of previous treatment for this episode.

B. *Physical examination.* (1) Temperature; (2) blood pressure; (3) palpation of abdomen with reference to suprapubic and CVA regions; (4) genitalia (external genital exam for females); (5) rectal (males only).

C. *Laboratory (in addition to quantitative urine culture).* Clean voided urine specimen for routine analysis and microscopic examination of sediment.

III. Management

A. *Criteria for treatment.* (1) Treat all patients with 100,000 colonies per ml of any pathogenic organism; (2) with symptoms of sepsis or bacteria on unspun urine sediment, treat prior to results of quantitative culture; (3) less than 10,000 colonies per ml of any organism and no history of previous treatment: no treatment indicated; (4) 10,000–100,000 colonies per ml of any pathogenic organism: require three positive quantiative cultures before treating.

B. *Hospitalization with initial infection indicated:* (1) If patient is acutely ill on presentation as indicated by presence of sepsis (fever, sweat, prostration, chills) or by being too ill to come to physician's office without help; (2) where obstruction is present as well as infection; (3) where infection accompanied by renal failure.

C. *Office treatment indicated.* The patient who is uncomfortable, but not septic, and can pass urine should be treated as an outpatient.

D. *Treatment.* (1) Symptomatic treatment for dysuria without evidence of bacterial infection; (2) antibacterial treatment.

All drugs are prescribed in acceptable dosages adjusted to the individual patient, contraindications are observed, and patients are monitored for common side effects according to information detailed in *AMA Drug Evaluations, 1971.* Fixed-dosage combinations should not be used for initial therapy.

Initial treatment with a soluble sulfonamide, tetracycline, ampicillin, or nitrofurantoin. If within 48 hours the symptoms do not respond to the first drug: alternative drug therapy should be initiated. Duration of antimicrobial treatment: 7–14 days.

E. *Follow-up.* (1) Repeat urine culture one week after treatment is stopped; (2) intravenous pyelogram (IVP) for history of infection during childhood, more than two episodes in females, and after first episode in males.

F. *Referral.* (1) To urologist if there is IVP evidence of genitourinary anomaly or obstruction; (2) to specialist for treatment of persistent and resistant bacterial infection in the absence of genitourinary anomaly or obstruction.

CLINICAL ASPECTS

Bacterial infections of the urinary tract are the second most common infections encountered in medical practice and can lead to serious acute and chronic disease.[1,2,3]

A clinical designation of urinary tract infection or bacteriuria relies on the detection of significant numbers of viable bacteria in the urine, with or without evidence of tissue reaction to these bacteria. The most widely accepted measure of significance is the quantitative colony count, established from observations by Kass[4,5] and confirmed by others.[6] More than 100,000 pathogenic organisms per ml of urine has come to be accepted as a reliable indication of the presence of a true infection.[7,8] Urine is considered contaminated at an organism count between 1,000 and 10,000 per ml of urine;[9] within the range of 10,000 and 100,000 organisms per ml, a culture is judged equivocal or inconclusive. For this review, significant bacteriuria, unless specifically noted, designates the presence of more than 100,000 bacteria per ml of urine in at least two consecutive specimens. The methods of urine collection and culture processing vary considerably and will be discussed below in more detail.

The organism most commonly detected in infected urine is *Escherichia coli.*[8,9] Other organisms responsible for urinary tract infections include *Klebsiella, Proteus, Pseudomonas, Enterococcus, Aerobacter, Staphylococcus,* and *Streptococcus.*

Bacteria may be present in abundance in the urine without evidencing any symptoms; as such, an infection may remain undetected and persist at a subclinical level for some time. Considerable evidence indicates that there are many more individuals suffering from undiagnosed chronic episodes of urinary tract infection than persons in whom it is clinically diagnosed. The presence of symptoms directly related to the urinary tract is more often the exception than the rule, emphasizing the chronic and insidious nature of the infection.[3,4,10]

When they exist, the symptoms, signs, and abnormal urinary findings associated with these infections are most often indicative of lower urinary tract infection. The clinical picture may include urgency and frequency of urination, initial or terminal dysuria, and sometimes fever. Infections of the upper urinary tract are often accompanied by costovertebral pain, nausea, vomiting, fever above 101 °F, and shaking chills.

METHODOLOGICAL CONSIDERATIONS

A review of the available literature highlights several methodological difficulties. These technical problems do not seriously impair the value of the data, but they do affect the bases from which any inferences, interpretations, and conclusions can be made. Because the following discussion is merely a brief overview of the most relevant issues, a detailed analysis of the clinical procedures and their comparable reliabilities are not presented.

The presence of bacteriuria is contingent on the diagnostic criteria and methods of both specimen collection and culture processing. Investigators have amply demonstrated that variations in these procedures critically affect the reported rates of bacteriuria.[2,3,4,6,7,11-14] Furthermore, the absence of standard criteria for such diagnostic entities as cystitis, pyelonephritis, and renal papillary necrosis makes it difficult to utilize data from studies that employ these labels. For this reason, a decision was made to concentrate this review on "significant bacteriuria," as quantitatively defined by the presence of more than 100,000 bacteria per ml of urine in at least two consecutive specimens without consideration of the anatomic site of infection.

It is more difficult to diagnose urinary tract infection in infancy, and especially in the neonatal period, than at any other age because of obvious problems in urine collection. Concern has also been expressed over the method used to obtain urine specimens from other age groups as well. The most widely accepted procedure has been the procurement of fresh, clean-voided ("clean-catch") specimens. Some investigators use voided specimens that have been collected by the patients themselves, while others use specimens collected by trained technicians. In women, a catheterization is often performed to avoid coincidental contamination from the vagina or introitus. At the level of 100,000 bacteria per ml of urine, some investigators maintain that a single catheterized specimen can be used with about 96 percent confidence, compared to two consecutive clean-voided specimens otherwise required in order to reach the same degree of confidence.[3,9,11] However, instrumentation is often suggested as a possible precursor to urinary tract infections, although the definite impact of a single straight catheterization remains in dispute. It has been suggested that not only may certain populations be in danger of postcatheterization infection, but also that this technique of urine collection yields higher rates, which can be attributed to either newly induced infections or better detection.[3,7,15−18]

Preparation of the patient, i.e., cleansing the external genitals and periurethral area, lends itself to procedural variation. Some investigators maintain that rates may be as much as 20 percent higher if the patient is not washed,[13] whereas others report that antiseptic cleansing may give rise to false negatives[19] if the antiseptic contaminates the collecting container.

The tendency of bacteria to multiply in the urine after sampling cannot be overlooked in this discussion. Although investigators vary in their estimates of postsampling changes,[4,11] there is a consensus that the time lapse between urine collection and culture process, the manner in which the specimen is stored, the medium selected to culture the urine, and the method used to enumerate the bacteria are all significant factors affecting the confidence limits of the bacteriologic findings.

The inability to define accurately the distribution of urinary tract infection among various population groups is due, in part, to lack of comparable samples and incomplete data reporting. The differentiation of populations as inpatient versus outpatient or clinic versus general is extremely important, especially with respect to available forms of diagnostic procedures and the overrepresentation of particular demographic groups. Unfortunately, information available on the frequency of urinary tract infection in the general population is derived mainly from hospital or clinic statistics, which tend to include disproportionate numbers of high-risk groups.

EPIDEMIOLOGY

AGE AND SEX

The literature documenting the prevalence and incidence of urinary tract infection suggests fairly consistent epidemiologic patterns with respect to both age and sex. Investigators concur that the frequency of bacteriuria generally increases with age for both males and females. Furthermore, available data indicate that the risk of infection is significantly greater for females than males at all ages, with the exception of the infant and geriatric years.

Because of the characteristically low frequency of urinary tract infection among men, very few studies have included males in their population samples. Therefore, in analyzing prevalence and incidence rates for age patterns, sex-related patterns should be delineated.

Studies based on neonatal and infant populations are rare, although existing data suggest that urinary tract infection constitutes one of the more potentially serious infections of this age group.[20-22] Available statistics are derived principally from hospital and outpatient populations, indicating that bacteriuria, though not uncommon in infants, is less common than in later years. Prevalence rates usually fall within the range of 0.3 and 7 percent,[23-29] although some studies report rates as high as 10 percent. Among apparently healthy infants rates as high as 30 percent have been noted; these extreme figures usually are attributed to perineal contamination,[24] but the precise explanation remains unclear. In general, significant bacteriuria is thought to occur 1.5 to 2.3 times more frequently in males than in females in the first year of life,[30] which can largely be attributed to congenital genitourinary anomalies.[27]

In a hospital survey of the National Maternity Hospital in Ireland, O'Brien and Dundon[26] find that the male is more likely to develop urinary tract infection in the first month of life than the female. In fact, over a 15-month period, no cases of infection were detected among female infants. The rate for both sexes is reported to be 1.6 percent on initial screening and 0.3 percent after a second specimen was cultured.[24] This data has been validated by Cahalane and Boothman.[31] Among infants under 12 months, 4.9 percent of the males versus 3.9 percent of the females have significant bacteriuria, yielding an overall prevalence rate of 4.5 percent. This rate is markedly higher than the overall prevalence rate reported by O'Brien and Dundon, suggesting the possibility of contaminated specimens. However, O'Brien and Dundon studied apparently healthy neonates, whereas Cahalane and Boothman considered infants hospitalized for a variety of reasons.

A few studies do not report a higher frequency of bacteriuria in newborn males. Forbes *et al.,*[32] for example, finds equal distributions with respect to sex and age in a study group of 90 children from a pediatric outpatient unit. However, there are only eight infants under 1 year of age in his sample.

The study by Randolph and Greenfield,[27] one of the few available surveys of infants in a private pediatric practice, indicates a greater frequency among female infants than males. However, the population under study lacks a representative number of infants between birth and 3 months, purportedly a high-risk age for males.

The frequency of urinary tract infection among preschool children has not been completely defined. However, the accumulated evidence indicates that the tendency for females to incur higher infection rates than males emerges during these years.[19,25,33] For example, Randolph and Greenfield[27] repeat the survey discussed above for the same children over a span of 13 months and find an increased sex differential: A period prevalence of 4.5 percent for females and 0.5 percent for males is recorded.

It should be noted that several studies of the preschool age group have emphasized that the lack or vagueness of symptoms may not alert the physician to the possibility of infection. In a population survey of 5-year-old girls, Savage et al.[19] determine a 2.1 percent prevalence for asymptomatic bacteriuria, indicating a critical number of previously undetected infections.

Recently, considerable attention has been directed toward establishing the prevalence of urinary tract infection in school children. The literature reveals a generally consistent trend with respect to distribution by sex, i.e., the frequency of infection is significantly greater for females than males. The trend continues for all subsequent age groups until the fifth decade.[2,3,11,12,17,30,32,34–56]

This pattern has been reported in the extensive series of epidemiologic studies conducted by Kunin and his associates in central Virginia.[8,20,38–41,57–59] Over a 10-year period, they screened thousands of asymptomatic children from public, parochial, and private schools, in grades one through twelve. The overall prevalence in the general population was 1.2 percent for girls and 0.03 percent for boys. One group of girls, studied six times over a period of 7 years, from age 6.5 to 13.5 years,[57] were found to contract new infections at the rate of 0.3 percent a year (Figure 1). Kunin interprets the cumulative rate over the 7 years to be 2.9 percent, although only about 1 percent of the girls were bacteriuric at any one time.

Based on his observations, Kunin draws the following conclusions:

1. All girls between the ages of 6 and 19 years are at equal risk for

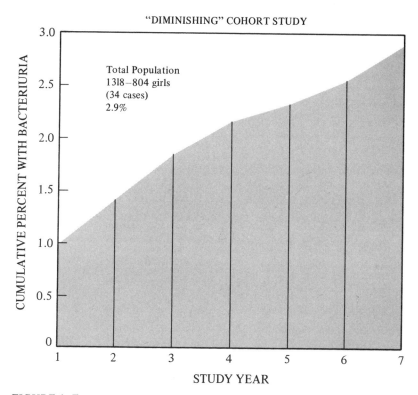

FIGURE 1 Emergence of bacteriuria among a sample population of girls studied on six occasions over 7 years. From Kunin CM: Epidemiology of bacteriuria and its relation to pyelonephritis. J Infect Dis 120:1–12, 1969. Copyright © 1969. Reprinted by permission of the University of Chicago Press.

acquiring bacteriuria at some point during these school-age years.[39]

2. The risk of infection for an individual girl decreases as her time without bacteriuria is extended, but each occurrence of infection predisposes the individual to subsequent episodes.[40]

As noted above, there is a consensus among investigators with respect to the frequency of bacteriuria during the school-age years, despite a few studies in which divergent results have been reported. For example, Bhagat *et al.,*[60] in a study of 500 girls and 500 boys between the ages of 5 and 11 in India, finds the overall rate of 1.8 percent to compare well to that observed by Kunin, but Bhagat and his associates do not report significant differences by sex. Cahalane and Boothman[31] find substantially higher overall prevalence rate of 2.4

percent, but their study population consisted of unselected hospital children and included high-risk infants and neonates. The overall prevalence is reduced to 1.4 percent when the population is restricted to children over age 5, and significant infection is almost entirely confined to females.

Information on the prevalence and incidence of urinary tract infection in adults is derived mainly from hospital statistics. Occasionally morbidity data are collected from general practices. It should be noted, however, that many surveys of general practices, outpatient clinics, and hospitals tend to include a disproportionate number of pregnant women. An attempt has been made to eliminate these studies from the present discussion, since their inclusion might seriously affect distribution rates in the general adult population. This purported high-risk population of child-bearing women will be discussed specifically in a later section.

Kass and associates[3,12,50,61] investigated the prevalence of bacteriuria in defined rural and urban populations of Jamaica and in mining and agricultural populations of Wales. The overall prevalence for 3,057 females was 4.4 percent with variations ranging from 2.2 to 4.9 percent for the different population groups. When analyzed in relation to age, the frequency of bacteriuria increases about 1 or 2 percent per decade, beginning with a rate of about 2 percent for females age 15–24 and reaching about 10 percent for females age 55–64 (Figure 2). Based on re-examinations of the Jamaican population, the number of spontaneous cures appears to equal the number of new infections.

Freedman et al.[35,62] studied approximately 3,000 women from general adult populations in Japan. Prevalence rates increased with advancing age, ranging from about 1 percent in women age 20–29 to about 3 percent in women age 50–59. These rates are similar to those reported in urban Jamaica, but lower than those reported in rural Jamaica and Wales.

Surveys of general-practice patients reveal slightly higher rates for urinary tract infection than those found in surveys of general adult populations. For example, Manners et al.[63] observe an overall prevalence rate of 8.5 percent for 720 women between the ages of 16 and 65. Tuxford[55] surveyed 19 general practices in Great Britain and reports an overall prevalence of 9 percent among 456 females, with variations among the practices ranging from 0 to 24 percent.

Studies based on hospitalized women demonstrate even higher rates of infection. Kass[4,64] observes significant bacteriuria in 30 percent of the women on the medical wards and only in 6 percent of the

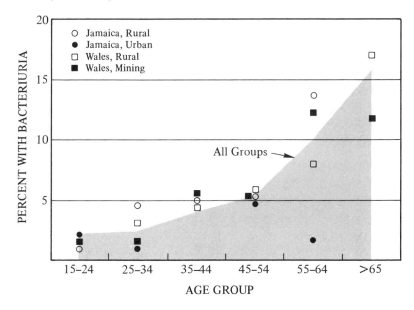

FIGURE 2 Prevalence of bacteriuria in relation to age in females of selected population groups. From Kass *et al.*[12]

women from the medical outpatient clinic at the Boston City Hospital. Kaitz and Williams[65] find that approximately 15 percent of women in a general hospital population had bacteriuria on admission. In an earlier study, Marple[66] discovers infections in 24 percent of women hospitalized in general medical wards. These higher rates found in hospital populations can probably be attributed to such factors as urinary tract instrumentation, concomitant illness, and general debility.

Epidemiologic studies reveal very low rates of bacteriuria in adult males selected from the general population. Kass and co-workers[3,12,50,61] report a prevalence rate of 0.5 percent for 1,515 males selected from the general population of Wales and Jamaica. In Japan Freedman *et al.*[35] do not observe bacteriuria at all in men under 50 and only in 0.6 percent of the men between age 50 and 59. Switzer[67] finds 0.2 percent of 427 males in Japan are infected.

The pattern of increased frequency of bacteriuria with age continues for the geriatric age group. There is considerable evidence that the prevalence of infection and severity of episodes are greater among the elderly than any other age group.[3,9,65] Some investigators report that during these later years sex-related differences appear to diminish.[68–70]

In the general adult population of Japan, Freedman *et al.*[35] demonstrate that, for women, the prevalence rates changed from 2.8 percent in the fifth decade to 7.4 percent for 60-year-olds and to 10.8 percent for women over 70. Although there are no infections detected in men under 50, the rates more than doubled for each successive decade after 50, with 0.6 percent for those 50–59 years of age, 1.6 percent for the next decade, and 3.6 percent for men over 70. In a survey of geriatric patients from a general practice in Great Britain, Brocklehurst *et al.*[68] find that the high incidence of bacteriuria occurs after 65 for women and after 70 for men. Furthermore, this study demonstrates no sex-related differences in rates after age 70. The prevalence of significant bacteriuria for females over 65, as well as for males over 70, was 20 percent. The literature indicates that not only are the elderly at highest risk but, as in all other age groupings, institutionalized and hospitalized geriatric patients are particularly at high risk.[14,65,70-72]

RACE

The relationship of race to the prevalence, incidence, and chronicity of urinary tract infection has not been completely defined. Very few studies have been designed for the purpose of interracial comparisons, and even fewer have attempted to control for possible relevant factors, such as socioeconomic status and age. Nevertheless, the consensus appears to be that race, in itself, is not a major determinant of morbidity rates.

Documentation of the frequency of infections with respect to race in the general population relies heavily on the studies conducted by Kunin and his associates.[8,20,38-41,59] Screening more than 8,000 school-age girls in three separate surveys (Figure 3), Kunin and Paquin[59] find that the overall prevalence rates for black and white females are not significantly different—1.2 percent for whites and 0.9 percent for blacks. However, differences become significant when the data are analyzed by age. Between the ages of 5 and 14, the prevalence rate for black girls is significantly lower than for white girls, with rates recorded at 0.5 and 1.2 percent respectively. Between the ages of 15 and 19, however, the frequency rates reversed: The rate for black girls rises to 3.5 percent, compared to 1.4 percent in whites. This rate for older black girls is not only significantly higher than the rate for whites of the same age, but also for both younger whites and blacks.

The data suggest that this group of older black girls is particularly

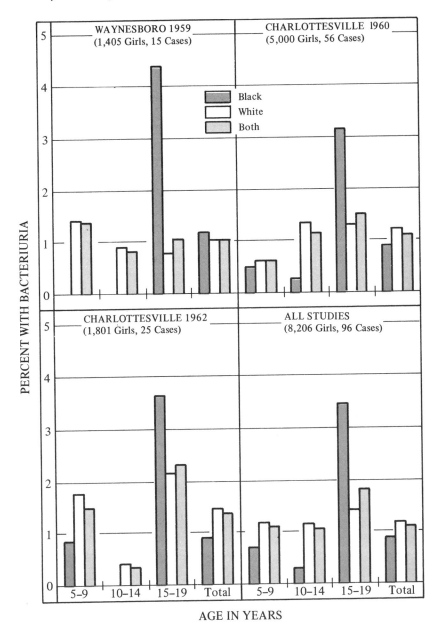

FIGURE 3 Prevalence of bacteriuria in schoolgirls, by age and race, as determined in three surveys. From Kunin and Paquin.[59] Reprinted by permission of F. A. Davis Co.

prone to infection. However, not only were urologic abnormalities rare in blacks, almost all cases of spontaneous cures occurred in that group. Furthermore, among black populations, recurrent infections are less common and tend to be delayed, especially after the first cure. Therefore, after considering other relevant rates, the authors[59] conjecture that urinary tract infection may actually be more common in whites.

Mou's[51] findings are essentially those described above. In addition to the qualifications suggested by Kunin and Paquin,[59] Mou notes that the sample of black women include a disproportionate number of pregnant women, supposedly a high-risk group.

Kunin and McCormack[73] compare the prevalence of bacteriuria among 2,882 white and 422 black nuns with 2,302 white and 390 black working women. The rates are virtually identical for white and black nuns, significantly higher for black than white working women, and generally more frequent for working women than nuns, regardless of race (Figure 4). The overall low rate of 1.9 percent among black nuns, versus the rate of 7.3 percent among black working women, again suggests that environmental rather than racial factors are determinant.

Many investigators have derived data regarding the distribution of bacteriuria with respect to race from studies of pregnant women. Turck et al.[74] conducted a prospective analysis of 1,727 pregnant women representing varying socioeconomic levels. Infections are significantly more common among black (8.6 percent) than white (2.7 percent) women in the total population. When analyzed by socioeconomic class, significant race differences are not observed among women of low financial, educational, and social status. Because less than 20 percent of the total black sample is not of low socioeconomic status, meaningful comparisons cannot be made for the upper-income group. Similarly, based on a study of 4,357 pregnant women all of low socioeconomic status, Whalley[56] does not observe significant differences among black, white, Latin American, and American Indian subjects. Norden and Kilpatrick[52] also find no correlation between bacteriuria and race in a hospital obstetric clinic.

A few studies of pregnant women, however, have documented overall significant differences with respect to race. Kaitz and Hodder[75] report 15.6 percent of black women and only 5.8 percent of white women have bacteriuria on their first visit to a hospital clinic. Henderson et al.[76] observe infections in 6.5 percent of black women and 2.5 percent of white women after routine catheterization at the time

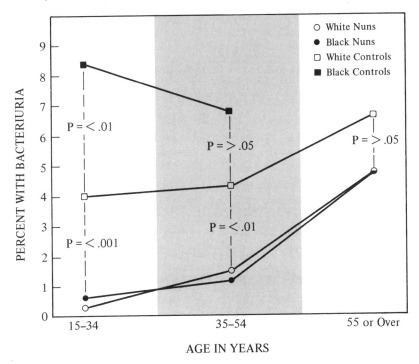

FIGURE 4 Prevalence of bacteriuria among nuns and working women, by age and race. From Kunin and McCormack.[73]

of delivery. The reason for these higher rates in some samples of black women is not clear. They may indicate a lack of adequate medical attention or other environmental factors indigenous to this population group. However, the different intraracial rates observed among black samples, in contrast to the comparable interracial rates documented between black and white samples of similar socioeconomic status, tend to eliminate the possibility of a racial predisposition to infection.

SOCIOECONOMIC FACTORS

Available epidemiologic studies have revealed an inverse relationship between morbidity rates and socioeconomic level, indicating that socioeconomic status is one of the more meaningful parameters in the distribution of bacteriuria.

The majority of investigators who have addressed themselves to these issues have based their studies on populations of pregnant

women. Williams *et al.*[77] conducted a study of pregnant women receiving prenatal care from a variety of sources in the city district of
Cardiff, Wales. A social class gradient operated at all age groups after
age 20 and at all parity groups (Tables 1 and 2). The occurrence of
bacteriuria was uncommon in women of high social class and increasingly more frequent among women of lower social status. Williams
and co-workers also find that women in lower-class groups have their
first child at younger ages than women in higher-class groups. These
investigators confirm the hypothesis that the younger the woman at
the time of her first pregnancy, the greater her risk of incurring bacteriuria. Multiparous women are the exception. Thus, it is inferred
that the influence of social class on frequency rates might be a function of age at first pregnancy.

Turck *et al.*[74] compare the prevalence of bacteriuria among pregnant women of different socioeconomic backgrounds by contrasting
women attending a county hospital with those attending private hospitals. The population from the county hospital is allegedly of low
financial, educational, and social background; the population selected
from the private hospitals is of middle-income and well-educated
status. Striking differences are observed between the two groups, with
overall rates reported at 6.5 percent for women attending the county
hospital and 2.0 percent for women attending the private hospitals.
For white patients, the prevalence rates are 5.1 and 1.9 percent for
county and private hospitals, respectively. There are too few black
women among the private patients to compare prevalence rates for
blacks, although blacks do demonstrate a higher rate than whites in
the county hospital. Turck and his associates conclude that women of
low socioeconomic status, especially black women, are at higher risk
than women in better circumstances. It should be noted, however,
that the cases of infection are detected by obtaining catheterized

TABLE 1   Standardized Bacteriuric Ratio by Age and Social Class

Social Class	Age (years)				
	Under 20	20–24	25–29	30 and Over	Total
1,2	–	0.86	0.65	0.86	0.68
3	1.44	0.87	0.84	0.94	0.94
4,5	1.07	1.52	2.26	1.11	1.51

Source: Williams *et al.*[77] Reprinted by permission of the Journal of Obstetrics and
Gynaecology of the British Commonwealth.

TABLE 2   Standardized Bacteriuric Ratio by Parity and Social Class

Social Class	Parity			
	1	2 and 3	4 and Over	Total
1,2	0.56	0.69	1.00	0.68
3	1.14	0.78	0.90	0.94
4,5	1.14	1.83	1.47	1.51

Source: Williams *et al.*[77] Reprinted by permission of the Journal of Obstetrics and Gynaecology of the British Commonwealth.

samples only at the time of delivery, allowing for the possibility of undetected infections and related or unrelated antimicrobial therapy during the course of the pregnancy. The investigators suggest that the differences observed between the population groups may be a result of disparities in the availability and use of such antimicrobial therapy.

As is the case with race, demonstration of the relationship between morbidity rates and socioeconomic factors in the general population relies heavily on the series of investigations of Virginia schoolgirls conducted by Kunin and his associates.[8,20,38,39,41,59] The level of education of both parents and the occupation of the father are used as measures of socioeconomic status. These indices, however, neither reveal any significant differences between the bacteriuric girls and the general population, nor indicate any social class distribution within the bacteriuric population (Tables 3 and 4).

It remains unclear whether socioeconomic differences in the prevalence patterns of bacteriuria are due to environmental factors or to disparities in both the availability of medical care and the use of antimicrobial therapy. Most investigators suggest that there is a greater tendency for individuals from higher socioeconomic levels to receive antibacterial treatment, often inadvertently curing infections of the urinary tract. Nevertheless, socioeconomic factors significantly affect the prevalence patterns of bacteriuria.

PREGNANCY

Surveys of a wide variety of populations have demonstrated that bacteriuria is one of the most common bacterial infections in pregnancy. The frequency of bacteriuria among pregnant women ranges from 3 to 9 percent (Table 5). Investigators concur that the frequency of bacteriuria generally increases with both age and parity.[13,38,52,56,74,]

TABLE 3 Comparison of Education of Fathers and Mothers of Bacteriuric Schoolgirls with that of Men and Women over Age 25 for Albemarle County, Virginia (1960 Census)

Educational Group[a]	Men and Women over 25 in County			Parents of Bacteriuric Schoolgirls		
	N	%	% Subtotal	N	%	% Subtotal
Male						
1	655	4.2		0	0	
2	1,981	12.6		5	3.7	
3	1,975	12.6		11	8.1	
4	1,407	9.0		8	5.9	
5	1,163	7.4		24	17.6	
			45.8			35.3
6	2,380	15.2		28	20.6	
7	2,130	13.6		28	20.6	
			28.8			41.2
8	1,187	7.6		6	4.4	
9	2,824	18.0		26	19.1	
			25.6			23.5
TOTAL	15,702	100.2		136	100.0	
Females						
1	404	2.4		1	0.7	
2	1,348	7.9		6	4.4	
3	2,014	11.7		9	6.6	
4	1,515	8.8		4	2.9	
5	1,205	7.0		14	10.3	
			37.8			24.9
6	2,922	17.0		43	31.6	
7	4,050	23.6		34	25.0	
			40.6			56.6
8	1,987	11.6		12	8.8	
9	1,704	9.9		13	9.6	
			21.5			18.4
TOTAL	17,149	99.9		136	99.9	

[a]Code: 1 = no school years completed; 2 = 1–4 years of elementary school; 3 = 5–6 years of elementary school; 4 = 7 years of elementary school; 5 = 8 years of elementary school; 6 = 1–3 years of high school; 7 = 4 years of high school; 8 = 1–3 years of college; and 9 = 4 or more years of college.
Source: Adapted from Kunin CM: Epidemiology of bacteriuria and its relation to pyelonephritis. J. Infect. Dis. 120:1–12, 1969. Copyright © 1969. Reprinted by permission of the University of Chicago Press.

[75,79,81,89–92] In fact, the correlation between age and parity is so high that it is often not possible to determine which of the two factors exerts a greater influence.[55,56,77,89] The younger the age of a woman at the time of her first pregnancy, the greater is her risk of incurring

TABLE 4 Comparison of Occupations of Fathers of Bacteriuric Schoolgirls with Those of Adult Men Reported for Albemarle County, Virginia (1960 Census)

Occupa-tional Group[a]	Adult Men in County		Fathers of Bacteriuric Schoolgirls	
	N	%	N	%
1	2,170	14.5	23	16.9
2	600	4.0	7	5.1
3	1,648	11.0	20	14.7
4	972	6.5	3	2.2
5	1,128	7.5	7	5.1
6	2,475	16.6	25	18.4
7	1,945	13.0	6	4.4
8	150	1.0	0	0
9	1,198	8.0	8	5.9
10	693	4.6	8	5.9
11	1,102	7.4	24	17.6
12	0	0	0	0
13	863	5.7	5	3.7
TOTAL	14,944	99.8	136	99.9
Father's Occupation group[b]				
I[c]	3,818	25.5	43	31.6
II[d]	6,520	43.6	41	30.1
III[e]	4,606	30.9	52	38.3
TOTAL	14,944	100.0	136	100.0

[a]Occupational code: 1 = professional, technical, and kindred workers; 2 = farmers and farm managers; 3 = managers, officials, and proprietros, except farm; 4 = clerical and kindred workers; 5 = sales workers; 6 = craftsmen, foremen, etc.; 7 = operatives, etc.; 8 = private household workers; 9 = service workers, except private household; 10 = farm laborers; 11 = laborers, except farm and mine; 12 = student; 13 = unemployed or unknown because mother unmarried.
[b]Donnelley et al.[78]
[c]Includes occupational groups 1 and 3.
[d]Includes occupational groups 4, 5, 6, and 7.
[e]Includes occupational groups 2, 8, 9, 10, 11, and 13.
Source: Adapted from Kunin CM: Epidemiology of bacteriuria and its relation to pyelonephritis. J. Infect. Dis. 120:1–12, 1969. Copyright © 1969. Reprinted by permission of the University of Chicago Press.

bacteriuria during that pregnancy.[19,77,79,86,87] Therefore, one finds an initial high risk associated with primigravid women under age 20. Lower morbidity rates are sometimes linked to the second pregnancy, with steady increases in rates usually accompanying each subsequent pregnancy.[49,52,77,79,87,92]

As discussed in the preceding section, Williams *et al.*[77] explicitly

TABLE 5   Frequency of Bacteriuria among Pregnant Women

Investigators	Number of Pregnant Females Screened	Bacteriuric (%)
Abramson et al.[79]	652	4.8
Bryant et al.[80]	448	7.1
Carleton et al.[81]	481	4.5
Carroll et al.[82]	5,200	6.4
Gold et al.[83]	1,281	5.1
Gruneberg et al.[84]	8,907	4.4
Hoja et al.[85]	1,000	4.9
Kaitz and Hodder[75]	616	4.4
Kass[3]	4,000	6.0
Kincaid-Smith et al.[6]	3,000	6.0
Leblanc and McGanity[49,86]	1,325	9.7
Little[87]	5,000	5.3
Monzon et al.[88]	1,400	7.3
Norden and Kilpatrick[52]	1,703	6.5
Savage et al.[89]	6,202	4.0
Stuart et al.[90,91]	2,713	3.5
Turck et al.[74]	1,727	3.4
Turner[92]	1,500	7.0
Whalley[56]	4,357	6.9
Williams et al.[77]	5,542	3.8

investigated the effects of age, parity, and social background as related to bacteriuria in a large-scale survey of an urban population in Wales. Based on over 5,000 pregnant women from hospital prenatal clinics, public health clinics, and a nursing home, this study provides one of the few available comparisons of the frequency of bacteriuria between age groups by parity (Table 6). A significantly higher rate is found among women under age 25 during their first or second pregnancy, but differences between age groups at higher parities are not significant.

When age at first pregnancy for bacteriuric women is compared with that for a control group of randomly selected nonbacteriuric women, 32 percent of bacteriuric women (but only 24 percent of the control group) have delivered their first baby before age 20. In addition, the bacteriuric rate decreases as the age at first pregnancy increases. This relationship is not as apparent among multiparous women (Table 7). Therefore, it is concluded that age at first pregnancy significantly influences rates among women at low parities: the younger the age, the higher the risk.

In summary, the evidence supports socioeconomic status, the cumu-

TABLE 6 Age/Parity Rates per 100 Women, Showing Significance in Age Group Rates within Each Parity

| Parity | Age | | | | |
	Under 20	20–24	25–29	30 and over	Total
1	5.1	4.8	1.8	2.0	4.1
2	4.7	5.7	1.7	3.4	3.8
		Under 25	25–29	30 and over	
3		2.9	2.4	2.8	2.7
4		2.9	5.1	2.7	3.5
		Under 30	30–34	35 and over	Total
5 or more		6.7	2.4	5.9	5.0

Source: Adapted from Williams *et al.*[77] Reprinted by permission of the Journal of Obstetrics and Gynaecology of the British Commonwealth.

lative relationship of age and parity, and the age at first pregnancy as factors that influence the frequency patterns of bacteriuria in pregnancy. The high-risk woman has been identified as being of low socioeconomic status and either multiparous and over 30 years, or primiparous and under 20 years.

OTHER ASSOCIATED FACTORS

Although very few investigators have addressed themselves to such environmental issues as geographic location and seasonal variation, the

TABLE 7 Bacteriuric Rate per 1,000 Women in Age and Parity Groups as Related to Age at First Pregnancy

| Age at First Pregnancy | Parity | | | |
	1	2 and 3	4 and more	Total
Under 20	51.1	51.2	42.0	49.4
20–24	47.7	31.8	49.8	41.2
25–29	17.9	21.9	21.9	20.4
30 and over	20.1	32.0	0.0	23.1
TOTAL	40.6	33.8	42.9	38.1

Source: Williams *et al.*[77] Reprinted by permission of the Journal of Obstetrics and Gynaecology of the British Commonwealth.

available literature does not suggest that the distribution of bacteriuria is meaningfully affected by either of these variables.[3,8,10,38,41,51,92] Currently, no significant differences in bacteriuric rates have been documented for even widely contrasting geographic areas. When slight variations in rates have been reported for different locations,[10,35,38,79] they have usually been attributed to factors other than geographical location, such as the nature and general availability of medical care.[11,41,74]

Only infrequently has the literature indicated seasonal variations in the distribution of bacteriuria. Mou[51] documents a tendency for lower rates in the fall and higher rates in the spring and winter, based on a relatively small sample population with a disproportionate number of pregnant women. Steensberg et al.[47] observe maximum frequencies during early summer and autumn. These seasonal distributions of bacteriuria are positively correlated with seasonal distributions of pregnancy, as derived from birth rates in the general population for the same area. Therefore, as with the influence of geographic location, any evidence of patterns of seasonal distribution probably can be attributed to the coincidental influence of other predisposing factors.

FUNCTIONAL IMPACT

Epidemiologic studies[93] of urinary tract infections document a graded risk of acquiring bacteriuria that varies with age in the female population. Kunin and his colleagues[20,42,59] report prevalence rates of about 1 percent in schoolgirls and estimate that 5 percent of girls will acquire bacteriuria during elementary and secondary school years.[49] Kass et al.[93] suggest that prevalence rates of bacteriuria rise by approximately 1 percent in women for each decade throughout life. The reasons for this continuous and graded risk are not understood; however, the magnitude of significant bacteriuria is emphasized by data[93] that indicate point prevalence rates for the total adult female population under age 65 to be 4–5 percent.

Investigations of the long-term effects of bacteriuria on renal structure and function, in general, document a decided risk of renal damage in the face of recurrent or persistent bacteriuria.[84,91] In a recent 10- to 14-year follow-up, Zinner and Kass[94] find radiologic evidence of pyelonephritis in approximately 30 percent of a small group of patients who had bacteriuria 10–14 years earlier, while none of the control patients had such abnormalities. Although there was incomplete follow-up of the total patient sample, these findings are consistent with the reports of other investigators.[56,95] In addition to the risk of pyelonephritis, bacteriuria does have deleterious effects on renal tubular function. Kaitz[96] demonstrates that renal concentrating ability is diminished in women with asymptomatic bacteriuria. Zinner and Kass[94] have recently published data with significantly lower mean maximal urinary osmolarity in patients with long-term bacteriuria than in comparable controls. Norden *et al.*[97] report that 14 percent of pregnant bacteriuric women cannot concentrate their urine, under maximal stimulation, above 700 milliosmoles.

Although the relationship of chronic pyelonephritis and hypertension has been studied intensively for over 30 years,[98] conflicting opinions exist.[99,100] Since the advent of quantitative urinary cultures, attempts have been made to study the association between hypertension and bacteriuria as one method of approaching this complex topic. In a study of a population of 428 hypertensive and 516 normotensive subjects, Switzer[67] is unable to demonstrate a relation between bacteriuria and hypertension. On the other hand, several investigators[73-93] have reported that persons with bacteriuria have tended to have higher blood pressure than nonbacteriuric. Kass *et al.*[93] suggest that their regression analyses are consistent with an association between bacteriuria and blood pressure that is independent of essential hypertension. These data are based on a small number of bacteriurics and as the authors suggest, "must be viewed cautiously."

As previously discussed, bacteriuria is a common complication of pregnancy, occurring in approximately 6 percent of pregnant women. It has been clearly demonstrated that if bacteriuria during pregnancy is untreated, approximately 20 percent will develop pyelonephritis later in pregnancy.[84] The reported incidence has varied from 14–63 percent.[56] Adequate chemotherapy of bacteriuria markedly reduces the rate of pyelonephritis, but does not completely eliminate it.[84]

Kass[13] was the first to indicate an association between bacteriuria during pregnancy and prematurity. Further, he suggests that eradication of the bacteriuria significantly reduced the risk of prematurity and fetal loss. This relationship has been studied by many investigators; some support Kass' findings[6,76] and others do not.[24,75,92] Kincaid-Smith and Bullen[101] confirm that there is an increased risk of prematurity in bacteriuric patients, but find that the prematurity rate is not influenced by successful treatment. The nature of this important relationship between bacteriuria and prematurity remains controversial.

A preliminary study[93] of mortality among bacteriuric persons has revealed that those with bacteriuria have an increased risk of death compared to those without. These data are based on a relatively small number of individuals and require further analysis and confirmation.

REFERENCES

1. Freedman LR, Epstein F: Pyelonephritis and infections of the urinary tract, Principles of Internal Medicine. Edited by TR Harrison, et al. New York, McGraw-Hill Book Co, 1966, pp 870–876
2. Kass EH: Renal and urinary disorders, Preventive Medicine. Edited by DW Clark, B MacMahon. Boston, Brown and Co, 1967, pp 539–552
3. Kass EH: Pyelonephritis and bacteriuria: A major problem in preventive medicine. Ann Intern Med 56:46–53, 1962
4. Kass EH: Asymptomatic infections of the urinary tract. Trans Assoc Am Physicians 69:56–64, 1956
5. Kass EH: Bacteriuria and the diagnosis of infections of the urinary tract. Arch Int Med 100:709–714, 1957
6. Kincaid-Smith P, Mullen M, Mills J, et al: The reliability of screening tests for bacteriuria in pregnancy. Lancet 11:64–65, 1964
7. Detection of bacteriuria. Lancet 2:71–78, 1964
8. Kunin CM, Deutscher R, Paquin A: Urinary tract infection in school children: An epidemiologic, clinical and laboratory study. Medicine 43:91–130, 1964
9. Petersdorf RG, Plorde JJ: Management of urinary tract infections in the elderly. Geriatrics 20:613–623, 1965
10. Waters WE: An epidemiological approach to urinary tract infections. J Infect Dis 120:136–150, 1969
11. Ronald AR: Urinary tract infection. Appl Ther 10:659–664, 1968
12. Kass EH, Savage WE, Santamarina BA: The significance of bacteriuria in preventive medicine, Progress in Pyelonephritis. Edited by EH Kass. Philadelphia, FA Davis Co, 1965, pp 3–10
13. Norden CW, Kass EH: Bacteriuria of pregnancy—A critical appraisal. Ann Rev Med 19:431–470, 1968
14. Wolfson SA, Kalmanson GM, Rubini ME, et al: Epidemiology of bacteriuria in a predominantly geriatric male population. Am J Med Sci 250:168–172, 1965
15. Gillespie WA, Linton KB, Miller A, et al: The diagnosis, epidemiology and control of urinary infections in urology and gynecology. J Clin Pathol 13:187–194, 1960
16. Levin J: The incidence and prevention of infection after urethral catheterization. Ann Intern Med 60:914–922, 1964
17. Stamey TA, Pfau A: Urinary infections: A selective review and some observations. Calif Med 113:16–35, 1970

18. Wren BG: Asymptomatic bacilluria. Associated factors. Med J Aust 1:802–805, 1970
19. Savage DC, Wilson MI, Ross EM, et al: Asymptomatic bacteriuria in girl entrants to Dundee primary schools. Br Med J 3:75–80, 1969
20. Kunin CM, Southall I, Paquin AJ: Epidemiology of urinary tract infections, a pilot study of 3,057 school children. N Engl J Med 263:817–823, 1960
21. Burke EC: Commentary on urinary tract infections in children. Mayo Clin Proc 40:113–120, 1965
22. Smallpeice V: Urinary Tract Infection in Childhood and Its Relevance to Disease in Adult Life. London, Heinemann Medical, 1968
23. Bergstrom T, Lincoln K, Redin B, et al: Studies of urinary tract infections in infancy and childhood. X. Short- or long-term treatment in girls with first- or second-time urinary tract infections uncomplicated by obstructive urological abnormalities. Acta Paediatr Scand 57:186–194, 1968
24. Gower PE, Husband P, Coleman JC, et al: Urinary infection in two selected neonatal populations. Arch Dis Child 45:259–263, 1970
25. Larkin VD: Asymptomatic bacteriuria and acute urinary tract infection in a pediatric population. J Urol 99:203–206, 1968
26. O'Brien NG, Dundon SP: Urinary tract infection in the newborn. J Irish Med Assoc 62:109–110, 1969
27. Randolph MF, Greenfield M: The incidence of asymptomatic bacteriuria and pyuria in infancy; a study of 400 infants in private practice. J Pediatr 65:57–66, 1964
28. Saxena H, Goswami P: Asymptomatic bacteriuria in infants and children. Indian J Pediatr 37:465–468, 1970
29. Smallpeice V: Urinary infection in the two sexes. Problems of aetiology. Lancet 2:1019–1021, 1966
30. Smellie JM: Acute urinary tract infection in children. Br Med J 4:97–100, 1970
31. Cahalane SF, Boothman R: Prevalence of urinary tract infection in hospitalized children. J Irish Med Assoc 62:362–364, 1969
32. Forbes PA, Drummond KN, Nogrady MB: Initial urinary tract infections. Observations in children without major radiologic abnormalities. J Pediatr 75:187–192, 1969
33. Deluca FG, Fisher JH, Swenson O: Review of recurrent urinary tract infections in infancy and early childhood. N Engl J Med 268:75–77, 1963
34. Etzwiler DD: Incidence of urinary tract infections among juvenile diabetics. JAMA 191:81–83, 1965
35. Freedman LR, Seki M, Phair JP, et al: Epidemiology of urinary tract infections in Hiroshima. Yale J Biol Med 37:262–282, 1967
36. El-Garhy MT: A pilot study on the prevalence of asymptomatic bacilluria in the school population of Assuit. Turk J Pediatr 9:156–160, 1967
37. Kelly DG, Duff F, Diskin SF, et al: Prevalence of urinary tract infection in Dublin school children. J Irish Med Assoc 62:420–422, 1969
38. Kunin CM: Epidemiology of bacteriuria and its relation to pyelonephritis. J Infect Dis 120:1–12, 1969
39. Kunin CM: The natural history of recurrent bacteriuria in school-girls. N Engl J Med 282:1443–1448, 1970

40. Kunin CM: A ten-year study of bacteriuria in schoolgirls: Final report of bacteriologic, urologic, and epidemiologic findings. J Infect Dis 122:382–393, 1970

41. Kunin CM, Zacha E, Paquin AJ: Urinary tract infections in school children. I. Prevalence of bacteriuria and associated urological findings. N Engl J Med 266:1287–1296, 1962

42. Lorber J: Chronic urinary tract infection in children. Curr Med Drugs 8: 15–29, 1968

43. Meadow SR, White RH, Johnston NM: Prevalence of symptomless urinary tract disease in Birmingham schoolchildren. I. Pyuria and bacteriuria. Br Med J 3:81–84, 1969

44. Mond NC, Gruneberg RN, Smellie JM: Study of childhood urinary tract infection in general practice. Br Med J 1:602-605, 1970

45. Pometta D, Rees SB, Younger D, et al: Asymptomatic bacteriuria in diabetes mellitus. N Engl J Med 276:1118-1121, 1967

46. Steele RE, Leadbetter GW, Crawford JD: Prognosis of childhood urinary tract infection: The current status of patients hospitalized between 1940 and 1950. N Engl J Med 269:883-889, 1963

47. Steensberg J, Bartels ED, Bay-Nielsen H, et al: Epidemiology of urinary tract diseases in general practice. Br Med J 4:390-394, 1969

48. Fry J, Dillane JB, Joiner CL, et al: Acute urinary infections. Their course and outcome in general practice with special reference to chronic pyelone-phritis. Lancet 1:1318-1321, 1962

49. Leblanc AL, McGanity WJ: A survey of bacteriuria in pregnancy, Progress in Pyelonephritis. Edited by EH Kass. Philadelphia, FA Davis Co, 1965, pp 58-63

50. Miall WE, Kass EH, Ling J, et al: Factors influencing arterial pressure in the general population in Jamaica. Br Med J 2:497–506, 1962

51. Mou TW: Bacteriuria in a "normal" family population, Progress in Pyelone-phritis. Edited by EH Kass. Philadelphia, FA Davis Co, 1965, pp 87–94

52. Norden CW, Kilpatrick WH: Bacteriuria of pregnancy, Progress in Pyelone-phritis. Edited by EH Kass. Philadelphia, FA Davis Co, 1965, pp 64–72

53. Silva Teles E DA, Rocha H: Bacteriuria in apparently healthy young adults. J Urol 102:342-344, 1969

54. Sussman M, Asscher AW, Waters WE, et al: Asymptomatic significant bacteriuria in the non-pregnant woman. I. Description of a population. Br Med J 1:799-803, 1969

55. Tuxford AF: Unsuspected urinary infection in general practice. JR Coll Gen Pract 20:22-26, 1970

56. Whalley PJ: Bacteriuria in pregnancy, Progress in Pyelonephritis. Edited by EH Kass. Philadelphia, FA Davis Co, 1965, pp 50-57

57. Kunin CM: Emergence of bacteriuria, proteinuria, and symptomatic urinary tract infections among a population of school girls followed for 7 years. Pediatrics 41:968-976, 1968

58. Kunin CM, Halmagyi NE: Urinary tract infections in schoolchildren. II. Characterization of invading organisms. N Engl J Med 266:1297-1301, 1962

59. Kunin CM, Paquin AJ: Frequency and natural history of urinary tract infec-

tion in school children, Progress in Pyelonephritis. Edited by EH Kass. Philadelphia, FA Davis Co, 1965, pp 33–44

60. Bhagat AK, Chouhan SS, Kaul KK: Incidence and nature of urinary tract infections among asymptomatic primary school children. Indian Pediatr 7:87–90, 1970

61. Kass EH, Miall WE, Stuart KL: Relationship of bacteriuria to hypertension: Epidemiological study. J Clin Invest 40:1053, 1961

62. Freedman LR, Seki M, Phair JP, et al: Proteinuria in Hiroshima and Nagasaki, Japan. Yale J Biol Med 40:109–140, 1967

63. Manners BT, Dulake C, Grob PR: Urinary tract infection in women: A study from general practice. J R Coll Gen Pract 19:343–348, 1970

64. Kass EH: Bacteriuria and the diagnosis of infections of the urinary tract. Arch Intern Med 100:709–714, 1957

65. Kaitz AL, Williams EJ: Bacteriuria and urinary tract infections in hospitalized patients. N Engl J Med 262:425, 1960

66. Marple CD: Frequency and character of urinary tract infections in an unselected group of women. Ann Intern Med 14:2220–2239, 1941

67. Switzer S: Bacteriuria in a healthy population and its relation to hypertension and pyelonephritis. N Engl J Med 264:7–10, 1961

68. Brocklehurst JC, Dillane JB, Griffiths L, et al: The prevalence and symptomatology of urinary infection in an aged population. Gerontol Clin 10:242–253, 1968

69. Paulett JD, Buxton JD: Pilot study of old-age pensioners. Br Med J 1:432–436, 1969

70. Walkey FA, Judge TG, Thompson J, et al: Incidence of urinary infection in the elderly. Scott Med J 12:411–414, 1967

71. Dontas AS, Papanayiotou P, Marketos S, et al: Bacteriuria in old age. Lancet 2:305–306, 1966

72. Mou TW, Siroty R, Ventry P: Epidemiology of bacteriuria among elderly chronically ill patients. Clin Res 9:174, 1961

73. Kunin CM, McCormack RC: An epidemiologic study of bacteriuria and blood pressure among nuns and working women. N Engl J Med 278:635–642, 1968

74. Turck M, Goffee BS, Petersdorf RG: Bacteriuria of pregnancy. Relation to socioeconomic factors. N Engl J Med 266:857–860, 1962

75. Kaitz AL, Hodder EW: Bacteriuria and pyelonephritis of pregnancy: A prospective study of 616 pregnant women. N Engl J Med 265:667–672, 1961

76. Henderson M, Tayback M, Entwisle G: Prevalence of significant asymptomatic bacteriuria and its association with prematurity in Negro and white women. Clin Res 9:202, 1961

77. Williams GL, Campbell H, Davies KJ: The influence of age, parity, and social class on the incidence of symptomatic bacteriuria in pregnancy. J Obstet Gynecol Br Commonw 76:229–239, 1969

78. Donnelly JF, Flowers CE Jr., Creadick RN, et al: Parental, fetal, and environmental factors in perinatal mortality. Am J Obstet Gynecol 74:1245–1254, 1957

79. Abramson JH, Sacks TC, Flug D, et al: Bacteriuria and hemoglobin levels in pregnancy. JAMA 215:1631–1637, 1967
80. Bryant R, Windom R, Vinyard J, et al: Asymptomatic bacteriuria in pregnancy and its association with prematurity. J Lab Clin Med 63: 224–231, 1964
81. Carleton HG, Baker TH, Richards AL: Bacteriuria in pregnancy. Am J Obstet Gynecol 92:227–231, 1965
82. Carroll R, MacDonald D, Stanley JC: Bacteriuria in pregnancy. Obstet Gynecol 32:525–527, 1968
83. Gold EM, Traub FB, Daichman I, et al: Asymptomatic bacteriuria during pregnancy. Obstet Gynecol 27:206–209, 1966
84. Gruneberg RN, Leigh DA, Brumfitt W: Relationship of bacteriuria in pregnancy to acute pyelonephritis, prematurity, and fetal mortality. Lancet 2:1–3, 1969
85. Hoja WA, Hefner JD, Smith MR: Asymptomatic bacteriuria in pregnancy. Obstet Gynecol 24:458–462, 1964
86. Leblanc AL, McGanity WJ: The impact of bacteriuria in pregnancy: A survey of 1300 pregnant patients. Tex Rep Biol Med 22:336–347, 1967
87. Little PJ: The incidence of urinary infection in 5000 pregnant women. Lancet 2:925–928, 1966
88. Monzon OT, Armstrong D, Pion RJ, et al: Bacteriuria during pregnancy. Am J Obstet Gynecol 85:511–518, 1963
89. Savage WE, Hajj SN, Kass EH: Demographic and prognostic characteristics of bacteriuria in pregnancy. Medicine 46:385–407, 1967
90. Stuart KL, Cummins GT, Chin WA: Bacteriuria, pre-eclamptic toxemia, and prematurity, Progress in Pyelonephritis. Edited by EH Kass. Philadelphia, FA Davis Co, pp 45–49, 1965
91. Stuart KL, Cummins GT, Chin WA: Bacteriuria, prematurity and the hypertensive disorders of pregnancy. Br Med J 1:554–556, 1965
92. Turner GC: Bacilluria in pregnancy. Lancet 2:1062–1064, 1961
93. Kass EH, Miall WE, Stuart KL: Bacteriuria in a defined population. Presented at the meeting of International Epidemiologic Association. Budva, Yugoslavia, August 28–September 4, 1971
94. Zinner SH, Kass EH: Long-term (10 to 14 years) follow-up of bacteriuria of pregnancy. New Eng J Med 285:820–823, 1971
95. Gower PE, Haswell B, Sidaway ME, et al: Follow-up of 164 patients with bacteriuria of pregnancy. Lancet 1:990–994, 1968
96. Kaitz AL: Urinary concentrating ability in pregnant women with asymptomatic bacteriuria. J Clin Invest 40:1331–1338, 1961
97. Norden CW, Levy PS, Kass EH: Predictive effect of urinary concentrating ability and hemagglutinating antibody titer upon response to antimicrobial therapy in bacteriuria of pregnancy. J Infect Dis 121:588–196, 1970
98. Longcope WT: Chronic bilateral pyelonephritis: Its origin and its association with hypertension. Ann Int Med 11:149–163, 1937
99. Smith H: Hypertension and urologic disease. Am J Med 4:724–743, 1949
100. Bell ET: Renal Disease. Philadelphia, Lea & Febiger, 1946
101. Kincaid-Smith P, Bullen M: Bacteriuria in pregnancy. Lancet 1:395–399, 1965

BIBLIOGRAPHY

AMA Council on Drugs: AMA Drug Evaluations, 1971. Chicago, American Medical Association, 1971
Management of urinary tract infections. Med Lett 12:49–51, 1970
Recurrent bacteriuria. Lancet 2:554–556, 1970
The Medical Letter Reference Handbook. Reprints of Special Issues of the Medical Letter. New York, Drug and Therapeutic Information, Inc., 1969

SEVEN

Cervical Cancer

SUMMARY

SERVICE FUNCTIONS

In the adult female population, cancer of the cervix is useful as a tracer for case-finding activities and general medical management. The standard Papanicolaou test is now complemented by reliable self-administered cell collection techniques, providing a useful tool for screening high-risk populations that obtain little medical care. The process of screening reflects the organization of the delivery system for case finding. Specialized skills in history taking and physical examination are required for proper diagnosis, as is appropriate use of consultants for follow-up care. This tracer provides an entry to the inpatient system and an opportunity to evaluate the coordination between inpatient and follow-up care after discharge.

CLASSIFICATION

The two most important microscopic forms of cervical cancer are squamous cell or epidermoid carcinoma (the most common form of the disease), and adenocarcinoma, which accounts for less than 5 percent of the cases. At present, there remains considerable dispute over the relationship between carcinoma *in situ* and invasive carcinoma.

EPIDEMIOLOGY

Age It is estimated that in America 9,400 women died from this disease in 1970. Mortality data from the United States show a steadily increasing rate from the youngest age group until a peak is reached at about age 55. From 1941–1943 to 1958–1960, age-adjusted mortality rates per 100,000 females for cancer of the cervix in New York State fell from 15.3 to 8.3 while the age relationships remained substantially unchanged. Generally, annual incidence increases with rising age, peaking in the fifth decade. Age-specific incidence rates derived from several large-scale screening surveys reveal the following: 8.7 per 100,000 at age 20–29; 45.4 at age 30–39; 69.5 at age 40–49; 83.2 at age 50–59; 74.9 at age 60–69; and 54.1 at age 70 and over.

Race and Ethnicity Data from a variety of sources indicate a higher risk of cervical cancer for blacks than whites. United States mortality figures of 1960 show 8.5 deaths per 100,000 for whites and 15.8 for nonwhites. Statistics from the National Cancer Institute indicate that in six American cities the ratio of incidence rates, black-to-white, varies from 1.2:1 to 2.5:1. Studies in Memphis, Tennessee, report rates for carcinoma *in situ* for both white and black women: The latter have substantially higher rates at the younger ages (under 49) and over 70 years of age. Jewish women have very low rates of cervical cancer. Haenszel and Hillhouse cite incidence rates of 4.7 per 100,000 for this group compared to 17.1 for other whites, 53.6 for blacks, and 109.8 for Puerto Ricans. These findings hold regardless of country of birth.

Marital and Sexual Factors Investigations by Dorn and Cutler and others have demonstrated a significant difference in incidence rates between single (19.0) and married white women (42.1). The critical sexual risk factors include early age at first coitus and multiple sexual partners, which correlate with early marriage and multiple marriages.

Socioeconomic Status Investigations in Dutch and Welsh towns find higher mortality rates in the lowest social classes. Rojel's study in Denmark shows much the same results, with cancer rates increasing consistently with decreasing socioeconomic status. Although numerous other investigations demonstrate similar findings, the pattern that emerges is one in which the behavior patterns and life styles associated with lower socioeconomic status correspond to those factors that define high risk, that is, earlier first coitus, multiple partners, poor hygiene, and failure to use obstructive contraceptives.

Other Factors   Analyses of circumcision status, penile hygiene, contraceptive practices, and venereal disease indicate that these factors are associated with cervical cancer. These variables are, however, also related to social status and sexual experience. At this time, considerable evidence suggests that the etiology of cervical cancer is linked to sexual experience.

FUNCTIONAL IMPACT

More than 23,000 women died in the United States from malignant neoplasia of the genital organs in 1967. Almost 57 percent of those deaths were due to a neoplasm of the uterus and over one-half of these uterine cancers were cervical in origin. Survival rates for patients with invasive cervical cancer increased from 1940 through 1964 but have remained relatively unchanged since. Survival is related to the stage of the disease, and there has been little change among patients with regional spread since 1950–1954. Whereas the 3-year survival rate for localized invasive cervical cancer was 85 percent (1960–1964), the survival rate for regional cervical cancer for the same time period was 52 percent.

The Department of Health, Education, and Welfare carrried out a cost-benefit analysis of uterine cancer in 1966 and estimated that in 1970 7,826 deaths would occur due to cervical cancer, with a total earnings loss of $318,754,000. Based upon screening and treatment cost estimates and time lost from work resulting from disability or death, net dollar benefits of massive screening programs were estimated. These calculations indicate that treatment of these cases at an early stage resulted in estimated net savings of over $60 million. Many assumptions that could be criticized, some based on tenuous data, are necessary to make these calculations. Nevertheless, the impact of cervical cancer is dramatized by the women-days lost.

A MINIMAL-CARE PLAN FOR CARCINOMA
OF THE CERVIX

I. Screening

A. *Papanicolaou smear (*PAP*).* (1) Any female having sexual intercourse regardless of age; (2) age 20 and over; (3) yearly or every 6 months if on oral contraceptives.

B. *Follow-up.* (1) Class I: repeat PAP at 1-year intervals for 3 consecutive years and then every other year thereafter; (2) class II: treatment of cervicitis if inflammation is present and repeat PAP in 3 months. If atypical cells ("atypia") are present, repeat PAP in 3 months. If dysplasia is present, repeat PAP immediately and then in 3 months; (3) class III: asymptomatic or symptomatic with or without lesion, refer to gynecologist for definitive histologic studies; (4) class IV or V: with or without lesion, refer to gynecologist for definitive histologic studies.

II. Evaluation

A. *History.* (1) Social: age at first intercourse; (2) Obstetrical: How many times have you been pregnant? (3) Menstrual: Are you still having menstrual periods? At what age did bleeding begin? Are they regular? Do you bleed between periods or after intercourse? Do you flow more than 7 days? Do you feel you bleed excessively? Have there been any recent changes in the amount of and/or length of time of your flow? (4) General: Are you doing anything to prevent pregnancy? Specify what contraceptive method. Do you have a vaginal discharge—Does it have an odor? Does it itch? What color is the discharge? Is it thick?—Have you had a PAP test (smear) in the past year? Have you ever been told you had an abnormal PAP?
B. *Physical examination.* (1) Pelvic and rectal examinations: describe external genitalia, vagina, cervix, corpus, adnexa, rectum.

Laboratory, treatment, follow-up and referral criteria are specified under Screening, B, points 1 through 4.

CLINICAL ASPECTS

The majority of carcinomas of the cervix are epidermoid or squamous-cell carcinomas that originate in the cervical canal. They account for approximately 95 percent of the histopathologic types, with adenocarcinoma and anaplastic varieties making up the remainder.[8]

Epidermoid carcinoma *in situ* (intraepithelial) is often a difficult pathologic diagnosis. The most important microscopic characteristics are epithelial hyperplasia, distortion of the architectural pattern, variation in size and shape of cells, and increased number of mitotic figures. These changes should be present through all layers of the mucosal surface, but contained within the mucosa, to permit the diagnosis of carcinoma *in situ*. The diagnosis of infiltrating or invasive carcinoma is made only when microscopic evidence of extension beyond the basement membrane is found.

Early in the course of the disease, the patient's only presenting symptom may be menstrual irregularities, often manifested by prolongation of the menstrual period. Minimal intermenstrual bleeding after coitus, exertion, or travel may be the first sign; hemorrhage— often the first symptom of advanced disease—on the other hand, rarely is associated with early lesions.

In the later stages of the disease, yellow vaginal discharge and bleeding are common. Weight loss and progressive lumbar pain with radiation to hip, thigh, and leg are almost invariably present with advanced disease. Accounting for many of these symptoms is the fact that carcinoma of the cervix spreads in three directions: to the fornices and vaginal wall; to the body of the uterus; and to the parametrium. Late symptoms are usually manifestations of secondary invasion of the bladder, rectovaginal septum and rectum, vulva, and uterosacral ligaments.

Metastatic spread is usually via lymphatics to iliac and hypogastric nodes with the sacral and lumbar nodes sometimes involved. Distant bloodborne metastases are not common from carcinomas of the cervix. The terminal event is often due to such complications as hemorrhage, bacteremia, peritonitis, or renal failure.

EPIDEMIOLOGY

High incidence rates for cancer of the cervix are found throughout the world.[1] In most western countries cervical cancer ranks second to breast cancer in frequency of malignancies.[2] A wide variation in incidence rates has been reported both within and between countries; an example of the range in rates is illustrated by Richard Doll's 1969 report in which annual incidence rates per 100,000 persons aged 35–64 years, standardized for age, varied from 14.8 in Israel to 247.3 in Cali, Columbia.[1] Data derived from large-scale screening surveys indicate that the annual incidence of cervical cancer for U.S. women

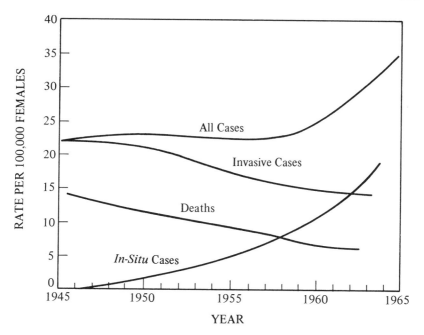

FIGURE 1 Cancer of uterine cervix death rates and incidence rates for New York State (except New York City), 1945–1964. From Porter *et al.*[6]

is between 37 and 44 per 100,000,[3,4] although higher rates are found in selected subpopulations. Prevalence rates for invasive and *in situ* carcinoma uncovered from mass screening efforts have been found to be 270 and 423 per 100,000, respectively.[5]

Examination of secular trends in incidence reveals contrasting patterns for invasive and *in situ* carcinomas. Figure 1 presents data from a study in New York State (exclusive of New York City) for the years 1945–1964.[6] A steady upward trend is seen for reported carcinoma *in situ,* while the incidence of invasive carcinoma is declining, especially after 1950. Deaths from invasive cancer also show a consistent decline since 1945 from approximately 14 per 100,000 to 6 per 100,000 in 1964.

More recent data based on sources compiled by the American Cancer Society reveal that the age-adjusted mortality rate from uterine cancer, mainly cancer of the cervix, had declined by one half in the last 30 years from 26.8 per 100,000 in 1935 to 11.1 per 100,000 in 1967.[7]

AGE

Data on the distribution of cervical cancer by age come from four sources: prevalence and incidence surveys, hospital case studies, cancer registries, and death records. The most accurate data are from mass screening surveys. Dunn et al.[9] couple their findings with the results of three other large-scale screening surveys and describe age-specific prevalence rates in white women for both carcinoma in situ and invasive carcinoma. For the latter, all four studies show an overall pattern of increasing prevalence with increasing age to age 70 (Table 1); maximum rates are generally observed in those women 60 years of age and older. These data are in contrast to Table 2 in which annual incidence rates for invasive carcinoma are given. Maximum incidence rates are reached about age 50 and then decline. This apparent discrepancy between Tables 1 and 2 is due to differences in the meaning of prevalence and incidence. Prevalence is defined as the number of cases at a

TABLE 1   Age-Specific Prevalence Rates for Invasive Cervical Cancer and Carcinoma in situ per 100,000 White Women as Determined in Four Studies and the Incidence of Clinically Evident Invasive Cervical Cancer in Memphis, Tennessee

Age Group (years)	San Diego	Charlotte, N. C.	Floyd County, Ga.	Memphis	Annual Incidence Rates of Invasive Cervical Cancer in Memphis
Invasive Cervical Cancer					
20–29	30	30	20	6	0
30–39	210	140	170	130	30
40–49	330	330	160	160	80
50–59	460	640	230	320	100
60–69	860	500	740	560	120
70 and over	250	1,640	740	730	140
Carcinoma in situ					
20–29	700	550	120(240)[a]	240	
30–39	1,150	700	280(450)[a]	480	
40–49	610	710	550(740)[a]	420	
50–59	710	440	300(600)[a]	280	
60–69	550	500	620(870)[a]	560	
70 and over	750	270	620(870)[a]	360	

[a]First figures designate "confirmed" cases. Rates in parentheses are sum of "confirmed" and "unconfirmed" cases.
Source: Adapted from Dunn et al.[9]

TABLE 2   Annual Incidence Rates of Invasive Carcinoma per 100,000 Females in Louisville and Jefferson County, Kentucky, and New York State (Exclusive of New York City), by Age and Specified Time Period[a]

New York			Kentucky	
Age Group (years)	1949–1951	1958–1960	Age Group (years)	1953–1955
20–24	2.2	4.9	20–29	8.7
25–29	8.7	16.9		
30–34	21.3	35.6	30–39	45.4
35–39	36.4	45.4		
40–44	50.4	58.7	40–49	69.5
45–49	56.6	53.6		
50–54	56.8	49.1	50–59	83.2
55–59	59.2	47.6		
60–64	58.4	42.7	60–69	74.9
65–69	63.1	48.1		
70–74	50.5	48.4	70 and over	54.1
75–79	58.6	44.7		
80–84	45.2	45.3		
85 and over	58.4	44.0		
TOTAL	27.4	26.5		51.4
Age-adjusted rate	25.2	25.9		33.8

[a]Adapted from Lundin *et al.*[10] and Stamler *et al.*[11]

given point in time within a defined population; incidence is the number of *new* cases developing over a given time period. Thus, prevalence is an accumulative measure and includes all individuals who survive the condition.

Carcinoma *in situ* has a different age distribution with a maximum prevalence at 30–39 years and no consistent trend with age. These generalizations hold true despite differences in the size of the population of the cited studies. For the most part these variations can be accounted for by differences in the study populations, type of cytologic specimen used, interpretation of borderline lesions, uniformity of specimens, and completeness of follow-up procedures.

Although the above data pertain exclusively to white females, the same author elsewhere reports prevalence rates for carcinoma *in situ* for black females. Negro rates were higher at the younger ages than for Caucasians: 440 per 100,000 at age 20–29; 691 at age 30–39; 591 at age 40–49; 223 at age 50–59, 438 at age 60–69, and 698 at age 70 and over.[5]

Data on the incidence of invasive carcinoma is not available for U.S. population as a whole. Reliance, therefore, is placed on regional data. Case registry reports submitted by physicians and hospitals in New York State, exclusive of New York City, have yielded incidence rates for two of these time periods, 1949–1951 and 1958–1960, are The age-adjusted incidence rates remain fairly constant over the three time periods: 25.3, 25.2, and 25.9 per 100,000, respectively. There is a noticeable downward shift, however, in age of highest incidence from age group 55–59 in 1941–1943 to ages 40–44 in 1958–1960. Stamler et al.[11] attribute this change largely to earlier diagnoses in the 1958–1960 period brought about by the introduction of the Papanicolau smear screening procedure. In Table 2 age-specific incidence rates for two of these time periods, 1949–1951 and 1958–1960, are compared with those derived from a 3-year morbidity survey in Louisville and Jefferson County, Kentucky, in 1953–1955. Although the age-distribution from the two sources follows the same general pattern, the rates from Kentucky are markedly higher for all ages above 29 years. This discrepancy may reflect the differences in data sources between the two studies, the New York data based on routinely reported, newly diagnosed cervical cancer cases and those from Kentucky on a large-scale screening program that probably uncovered asymptomatic pathologic states.

Unlike morbidity, mortality from cancer of the cervix does not level off or decline after age 59. United States mortality figures show a steadily increasing rate from the earliest age groupings until a peak is reached after age 65.[11] Similarly, the New York data presented in Table 3 point out a similar trend with mortality rising with increasing age.[11] While the overall age distribution has remained relatively constant for the three successive time periods studied, there has been a general decline in deaths at all ages, except the oldest group.

RACE AND ETHNIC GROUPS

Black Women   Data from a variety of sources indicate that blacks have higher rates of cervical cancer than whites.[12–14] United States mortality figures for 1960 show 8.5 deaths per 100,000 for whites and 15.8 per 100,000 for nonwhites (Table 4), a relationship that holds at all age levels. Statistics from the National Cancer Institute also indicate higher incidence rates for the Negro population (Table 5).

TABLE 3 Mortality Rates per 100,000 Females for Carcinoma of the Cervix Uteri, New York State (Exclusive of New York City), by Age and Specified Time Period

Age Group (years)	Time Period		
	1941–1943	1949–1951	1958–1960
20–24	0.00	0.39	0.14
25–29	1.84	2.14	1.11
30–34	5.04	4.94	3.99
35–39	15.62	9.94	6.96
40–44	21.46	16.09	11.94
45–49	30.76	26.71	15.88
50–54	31.21	29.23	21.26
55–59	44.94	32.86	20.17
60–64	45.33	29.73	21.24
65–69	49.16	40.35	27.72
70–74	57.19	41.76	33.92
75–79	59.32	59.14	28.01
80–84	63.34	44.35	37.33
85 and over	35.22	45.76	40.85
TOTAL	16.62	13.58	9.09
Age-adjusted rate	15.25	12.19	8.34

Source: Stamler *et al.*[11]

TABLE 4 United States Mortality Rates per 100,000 for Carcinoma of the Cervix Uteri, by Age and Race, 1960

Age Group (years)	White	Nonwhite
20–24	0.3	0.6
25–44	6.3	16.5
45–64	18.8	48.0
65 and over	27.8	56.5
20–64	10.5	27.8
All ages	8.5	15.8

Source: Stamler *et al.*[11]

TABLE 5 Incidence of Invasive Cancer of the Cervix per 100,000, 1947

City	White	Negro	Relative Risk Negro-to-White
Chicago	28	64	2.5:1
New Orelans	59	72	1.2:1
Dallas	44	65	1.5:1
Birmingham	52	73	1.4:1
Detriot	37	54	1.5:1
Philadelphia	33	65	2.0:1

Source: Graham et al.[15]

Analyses by Dunn et al.[14] in Memphis and Shelby County, Tennessee, have demonstrated an age-adjusted incidence rate for black women 1.7 times that of white women—64.1 and 37.6 per 100,000, respectively. Similarly, a 1952 survey of hospital admissions in New York City reveals an incidence rate for blacks 50 percent higher than for whites.[12] Although age-specific incidence rates rise with age for the black woman, these rates are higher at all ages than for her white counterpart (Table 6). These differences hold for both in situ and invasive carcinoma.[12,16,17] Figure 2 presents age differences between blacks, white non-Jews, and Jews. At age 30 black women have rates that approximate those for 50-year-old white women. The rates for blacks appear to peak at two points with a rate of nearly 118 per

TABLE 6 Annual Incidence Rates of Invasive Cervical Cancer per 100,000 Females in Louisville and Jefferson County, Kentucky, 1953–1955, by Age and Race

Age Group (years)	White	Nonwhite	Total
20–29	8.1	13.0	8.7
30–39	44.3	52.6	45.4
40–49	62.8	109.4	69.5
50–59	74.3	139.8	83.2
60–69	65.2	138.8	74.9
70 and over	46.4	119.8	54.1
TOTAL	46.5	84.3	51.4
Age-adjusted rate	30.7	54.3	33.8

Source: Lundin et al.[10]

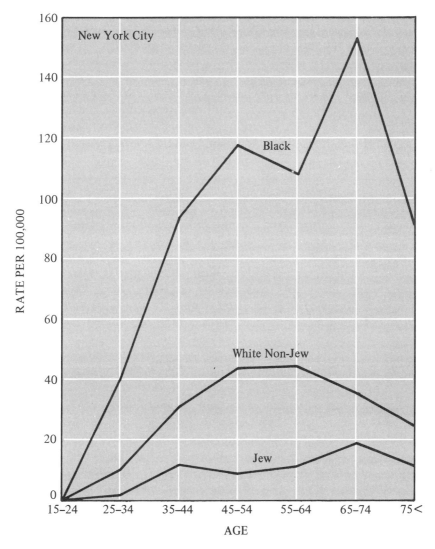

FIGURE 2 Incidence rates of invasive cancer of the uterine cervix, by age, in New York City, among blacks, non-Jews, and Jews. From Dunham.[17]

100,000 for the 45–54-year age group and approximately 150 per 100,000 in the 65–74-year age group, after which a decline is seen. The explanation for this bimodal curve in black women is not clear; however, it is possible that the late peak is a reflection of lack of early care resulting in detection at a later age when the condition is apparent. The white non-Jew shows a consistently lower rate at all ages and less variation with age.[17]

Jewish Women   The low rate of cervical cancer in Jewish women was first noted in 1901 by Braithwaite.[19] Vineberg, in analyzing data from Mount Sinai Hospital in New York City for the study period 1893–1906, gives these findings additional support.* In London, Austria, Hungary, Holland, Sweden, and Israel, statistics have repeatedly verified a low cervical cancer rate for Jewish women.[19]

In a study of hospital admissions over an 18-year period, Hochman *et al.*[21] discover an incidence rate of 2.2 per 100,000 Jewish women in Israel. Observations by Haenzel and Hillhouse[12] present similar findings giving comparative incidence rates per 100,000 of 4.7 for Jewish, 17.1 for other white, and 53.6 for Negro women.

Many theories have been offered to explain the low rates of cervical cancer among Jews. Socioeconomic variables, marital and coital practices, hygienic factors, circumcision status, genetic differences, and low penile cancer rates are most frequently associated with varying rates of cervical cancer. Each of these will be examined in detail later in the paper.

American Indians   American Indians, in particular, the Navajo, have been found by some to have a low rate of cervical cancer. A screening survey conducted by Jordan *et al.*[22] reveals that Pueblo and Navajo women have less than one half the prevalence of cervical cancer (330 per 100,000) as compared to non-Indian controls (790 per 100,000). In an earlier screening survey, Salisbury *et al.*[23] compare their rates showing invasive cervical cancer cases among Navajo women to that of a similar survey conducted among the total female population in Floyd County, Georgia, that finds morbidity to be 280 per 100,000. Indians in the Northwest, however, do not exhibit the same low rates as do those of the Southwest. Sheehan† finds a rate of 1,860 per 100,000 among northwestern Indians. Canadian Indians, too, have the disease 10 times more frequently than whites of that country.

Other Groups   Low rates of cervical cancer among various specific, religious subgroups have been noted in the United States. A screening study conducted among an Amish population in Ohio shows that this

* Cited in Lundin *et al.*[20]
† Cited in Jordan *et al.*[22]

group had only 108 cases per 100,000 examined as opposed to 527 cases per 100,000 non-Amish.[24] Two other sources cite low risk of the disease for Seventh-Day Adventists.[25, 26]

Similarly, studies of Roman Catholic nuns show consistently low rates of cervical cancer. Gagon[27] finds that the medical files of 13,000 nuns show no cases of cervical cancer. Records from other religious orders also show no evidence of the disease, although hospital pathology records do report confirmed cases among nuns.[27] A review[28] of mortality in three Catholic religious orders confirms these findings.

GEOGRAPHIC DISTRIBUTION

Cervical cancer rates are highest in the South and in urban areas. Haenszel and Hillhouse[12] studied newly diagnosed hospital admissions and discovered an age adjusted incidence rate of 17.1 per 100,000 white non-Jews in New York City. These same authors cite the contrasting rate of 49.5 described by Dorn and Cutler[3] for four southern cities. Nonwhites show less North–South variation than do whites, but this has been explained by the northern migration of many southern Negroes.[12] A comparable trend for mortality has been noted in the South, with more deaths from the disease in that region than in the North.

Data from hospitals, physicians' records, and formerly unreported cancer deaths in Iowa during 1950 show a difference in age-adjusted incidence rates in rural and urban areas of 23.6 and 43.4 per 100,000 women, respectively.[4] The variations noted were not found to be attributable to a difference in medical care or to underreporting of cases. A similar urban–rural pattern has been found in Denmark. Based on cancer registry data, Danish rural areas in 1954–1947 had rates half that of the average for Copenhagen.[29] As in Iowa, there is a high quality of care and diagnostic procedures in rural areas, so that the difference in rates is not believed to be due to lack of notification of cases.

SOCIOECONOMIC FACTORS

The relationship between socioeconomic status and the morbidity and mortality of cervical cancer has been well established. In general, most investigations reveal an inverse relationship between these factors. Stocks[30] compares cervical cancer mortality in a number of British and Welsh towns. Using the Registrar General's statistics, he observed higher mortality rates in towns with larger numbers of households in the two lower social classes.

Rojel's[31] study of syphilis and carcinoma of the cervix shows much the same results as the above. Cervical cancer rates increase consistently with decreasing socioeconomic status. Another Danish study, which agreed with these findings, uses rent paid as a measure of socioeconomic status.[29]

Lundin et al.[20] find what they consider to be a definite association between cervical cancer rates and socioeconomic status for whites in Memphis. Based on occupational criteria they discover an excess of cases in the lower status group. When they analyze their findings by income level, they discover a diminished association with suspicious cytological findings and intraepithelial cervical carcinoma. Age at first pregnancy is found to be earlier among the lowest socioeconomic group, but it only partially accounts for the excess of cases observed in this group. Dorn and Cutler[3] also find an inverse relationship between socioeconomic status and cervical cancer based on income.

Cohart's[32] study of New Haven, Connecticut, is the only report in conflict with the above findings. He divides the city into 24 ecological districts, grouping them into 7 socioeconomic areas and, more broadly, into 3 socioeconomic regions. There are no statistically significant correlations between incidence and socioeconomic area of residence. These findings may, in part, be explained by the relatively narrow range of social class in New Haven and the use of grouped socioeconomic data based on Census tract classification.

Table 7 shows findings from the U.S. 10-city survey (1947), as well as data from England, Wales, and Denmark, based on income class, Data presented are the ratios of observed to expected cases based on age and income specific rates. The results demonstrate that in each of the four countries, fewer than expected cases are seen in the higher strata groups 3, 4, and 5.

At this time, the available data strongly suggest that the inverse relationship between measures of socioeconomic status and cervical cancer rates are associated with a third set of variables—sexual practices.

ETIOLOGICAL CONSIDERATIONS

Many variables have been analyzed as possible etiologic factors in cervical cancer. Early marriage, early first coitus, parity, sexual prac-

TABLE 7 Standard Cervical Cancer Incidence Ratios, by Income Class for White Females in the United States, Denmark, England, and Wales

Class[a]	United States	Denmark	England	Wales
1	156	131	150	130
2	113	100	109	106
3	90	79	98	99
4	85	90	69	78
5	74	50	61	65

[a]1 is low and 5 is high.
Source: Dorn and Cutler.[3]

tices, hygiene, circumcision, contraception, and venereal disease are among the aspects most commonly considered. Available research on each of these factors has been reviewed and is discussed in relation to the demographic material previously presented.

Marriage and Sexual Practice Investigations by Dorn and Cutler[3] demonstrate a significant difference in incidence rates between single (19.0 per 100,000) and married (42.1 per 100,000) whites, and their data are supported by similar findings of other investigators,[25, 33, 34] Age of marriage has also been shown to be a significant determinant of risk,[13, 25, 35] with patients who married at younger ages having markedly more suspicious cytologic findings and cervical carcinoma than those who married later.[36]

Separation and divorce also have been observed more frequently in patients than in controls, as is seen in studies by Lombard and Potter[33] and Boyd and Doll.[34] With the high frequency of divorce and separation among patients, these women are more likely to have multiple marriages and multiple partners. This premise has been borne out in studies done by Wynder[37] and in two studies done by Terris[35, 38] and corroborated by Martin[26] and Rotkin.[39]

Specific sexual practices have been studied in relation to the onset of cervical carcinoma. Boyd and Doll[34] studied frequency of coitus between controls and patients and discovered that while cervical cancer patients had intercourse more often each month, the higher cancer rates were a function of their earlier age at first marriage. After standardizing for this variable, no differences were found between the two groups. Similar data have been reported by Jones *et al.,*[13] Rotkin and King,[40] and Rotkin.[39] Aitkin-Swan and Baird[41] and Rotkin[39] concur when they indicate that there appears to be a mean latency period of about 30 years between first coitus and first attendance for treatment of the disease.

In a hospital-based interview study of cervical cancer patients, a difference in age at first coitus is found between patients and controls, with 53 percent of patients and 26 percent of controls having a history of intercourse before age 17.[35] Terris and Oalmann, using gynecological controls and patients with cervical carcinoma from four New York hospitals, find 51.9 percent of patients and only 36.7 percent of controls[38] had first coitus before 17. In a carefully controlled study Rotkin emphasizes that early first coitus is a key risk factor.[39]

Most investigators agree that earlier age at first coitus is partially responsible for the high rates of cervical cancer among blacks. In their 10-city survey, Dorn and Cutler[3] attribute their findings of similar incidence rates between married and unmarried nonwhites—75.4 and 72.2 per 100,000, respectively—to similarities in their sexual practices. Haenszel and Hillhouse,[12] however, do find a lower rate among never-married nonwhites—27.7 per 100,000—than among married (or once-married) nonwhites—57.5 per 100,000. Racial differences seen in New York have been attributed to earlier coitus and higher remarriage rates among blacks, according to Terris and Oalmann.[35] These data are strengthened by a large-scale cancer detection program in which Negroes are found to marry, on the average, 3 years earlier than Caucasians.[42] However, Dunham's New York study[17] raises some questions about the role of early age at first coitus. Her data show that relatively more cancer patients than controls reported age at first intercourse between 14 and 17. However, this relationship is not found for first coitus under age 14 or at ages 18 and 19. Indeed, the median age at first intercourse of Negro patients with cancer of the cervix was 15.8, which is similar to the age at first coitus of an Israeli population with one tenth the incidence of cervical cancer as blacks.[17]

However, some investigators feel that the low incidence of cervical cancer observed among Jewish women is partially resolved by marital and coital factors. Most data indicate that Jewish women of today tend to marry at later ages than those of other populations. Wynder's[25] study of Jewish controls shows generally later age at first coitus and at marriage when compared to non-Jews, both white and black patients and controls. He concludes that this factor is at least partially responsible for their lower rates of cervical cancer. Data from Iowa also show a higher median age at first marriage among Jews, although it is felt that the difference between Jewish and other white women in age at first marriage is not great enough to account for the large difference in rates of cases between the two groups.[4] In a home interview study of Jewish patients and controls, Martin[26] discovers that such factors as coitus before age 20, early marriage, and broken marriages show the predicted excess among Jewish patients. This suggests that the same etiological factors are at work among Jewish women as among other whites and nonwhites. Findings from Israel support those from Martin's study. A high relative risk is noted for Jewish women marrying before the age of 20. However, no such excess risk is found among Jewish women from New York City marrying before age 20.[43]

The large number of women who have had a variety of sexual partners among cervical cancer patients gives rise to speculation on the part of some that risk of this disease increases as more partners are encountered. Rojel's[31] study in Denmark shows that out of 1,262 cervical cancer cases and 1,392 controls, there are four times as many prostitutes in the former group as in the latter.

Research based on a population screening of a Detroit detention home with matched controls from a Planned Parenthood clinic shows higher rates of gonorrhea, syphilis, and trichomoniasis in the prison group. The prison group also has much higher rates of abnormal cytologic findings. Coitus at an early age is extensive among patients. Moghissi *et al.*[42] suggest that the variables responsible for high venereal disease rates are the same as those that cause high cervical cancer rates, i.e., frequent sexual activity at an early age and multiple partners.

Considerable evidence thus indicates that the etiology of cervical cancer is somehow linked to sexual experience. The preponderance of this disease in married women and its deficit in nuns and celibate women point to this fact. The sexual variables discussed appear to be associated with other factors, including socioeconomic status, that partially define the behavioral characteristics of high-risk groups: early coitus and multiple sexual partners, variables strongly associated with early marriage, early dissolution of marriage, and multiple marriages. Parity, hygiene, circumcision, and concomitant diseases are additional factors that epidemiologic analyses have implicated as relevant to the etiology of this condition.

Parity Although cervical cancer can occur in the nulliparous,[44] data from England and America support the finding that cervical cancer patients are more likely to be parous.[15,45,46] Stocks[30] finds an association between cervical cancer patients and high fertility rates for those who married after 25. He attributes any connection between family size and the disease to environmental conditions that are frequently associated with high fertility. Aitken-Swan and Baird[41] interview subjects selected from a mass screening program and find three times as many patients with preclinical cancer as controls who have one or more pregnancies, including abortions, before marriage. This same high rate is found in patients with clinical cancer of the cervix. Coitus and pregnancies prior to marriage and the attendant socioeconomic implications are viewed by Aitkin-Swan and Baird as being of more importance than age at first marriage in accounting for differences in cervical cancer rates between patients and controls. In this same study, age differences are found to vary with the number of pregnancies, with the discovery of preclinical cancer rising to a peak between ages 45 and 59 in women who have 1–4 births. With five or more pregnancies, rates are highest in younger age groups and fall with advancing age. The large families seen among many cervical cancer victims are attributed to the same variables mentioned by Stocks[30] — socioeconomic status and life style.

Macklin's[47] findings agree in part with those of Aitken-Swan and Baird. In comparing women with and without cancer of the cervix, she finds that an excess number of cervical cancer patients are married and that among married women, cancer patients begin their childbearing at an early age and have large families. Cervical cancer patients have their first and second pregnancies an average of 7 and 5 years earlier than controls of comparable parity. Macklin's data suggests that age at first pregnancy is the most important factor.

Differences between nulliparity and parity in black patients and controls are observed by Dunham.[17] A large number of patients are found to have been pregnant. In addition, an excess of first pregnancy at ages 14–17 and a slight excess of patients having five or more pregnancies are noted. Dunham views age at first intercourse and early age at first and last pregnancy as interrelated factors typical of the behavior pattern mentioned above.

Venereal Disease   Syphilis is a disease frequently found concomitant with cervical cancer. Rojel's[31] extensive study based on hospital data from the Radium Centre in Denmark discovers 13.2 percent of 1,262 cervical cancer patients have syphilis, while only 4.1 percent of the 1,392 controls have the disease. An excess of syphilis is found among all social classes of cervical cancer patients. Rojel concludes that a relationship exists, independent of socioeconomic distribution, between the two morbidity conditions. At Roswell Park Memorial Institute, Graham *et al.*[15] finds 5.6 percent of 4,555 cervical cancer cases with syphilis, but concludes that this rate was only evidence of the behavior and socioeconomic status of the patient. These data do not support a causal relationship between syphilis and cancer of the cervix, although similar etiological factors may be at work in both conditions.[15] An analysis of cancer reports from New York State shows three times as many cervical cancer cases have syphilis as do women who have cancer of other sites (Table 8). Even controlling for marital status, the prevalence of syphilis among patients still remains high. Wynder[25] finds twice as much syphilis among white non-Jewish cervical cancer patients as among controls, but no such differences are found among Negroes. He feels, however, that earlier age at first coitus seen in cervical cancer patients can account for increased syphilis risk.

Contraception There is no clear-cut evidence that contraceptive practices vary significantly between cervical cancer patients and controls. Several studies do indicate that more controls than patients use obstructive contraceptive devices such as a condom or cap.[40,41,49] On the other hand, other investigators have found no differences re-

TABLE 8 Syphilis Prevalence among White Females with Reported Cancer of the Uterine Cervix and of Other Sites, by Age, in New York State (except New York City), 1940–1941

Age Group (years)	Cervix Cancer			Other Cancer			All Cancer		
	No. of Cases	Syphilis		No. of Cases	Syphilis		No. of Cases	Syphilis	
		No.	%		No.	%		No.	%
0–24	1	0	0.0	80	0	0.0	81	0	0.0
25–34	75	1	1.3	123	0	0.0	198	1	0.5
35–44	181	14	7.7	381	6	1.6	562	20	3.6
45–54	294	8	2.7	825	11	1.3	1,119	19	1.7
55–64	219	8	3.6	995	18	1.8	1,214	26	2.1
65–74	125	3	2.4	848	6	0.7	973	9	0.9
75 and over	35	2	5.7	428	0	0.0	463	2	0.4
All ages	930	36	3.9	3,680	41	1.1	4,610	77	1.7

Source: Levin ML, Kress LC, Goldstein H: Syphilis and cancer. NY J Med 42:1737–1744, 1942. Reprinted by permission from the *New York State Journal of Medicine*, copyright by the Medical Society of the State of New York.

garding contraceptive practices in the respective populations studied.[13,25,33] In a study of contraceptive practices and cervical cancer cases in New York, which included cytologic screening, a higher prevalence rate for cervical cancer *in situ* is found among those women who used oral steroids as their means of family planning. It would seem, however, that contraception is not as important as age at first coitus, marriage, hygiene, and parity.

Circumcision and Penile Hygiene   Circumcision is considered a means toward penile hygiene. With the foreskin removed, bacteria formation is less likely. The hypothesized carcinogen, smegma, has been shown in some studies to cause malignant neoplasma in mice. When Pratt-Thomas *et al.*[50] injected mice with biweekly doses of human smegma a significant number of carcinomas resulted. Wynder finds an increased risk for women with uncircumcised husbands, but tempers his conclusions by the fact that his study had a large sampling error.[25] Terris and Oalmann,[35] however, have also reported a higher proportion of patients than controls with uncircumcised husband. Testing for another variable—age at first coitus—and keeping circumcision status constant, Rotkin[39] finds that whether or not a woman has contact with a noncircumcised male does not affect the increase in risk associated with earlier onset of coitus.

Dunn and Buell[51] extensively analyze circumcision status based on interviews with cervical cancer patients and matched controls. The findings reveal no association between cervical cancer and lack of circumcision of the husband. However, the study is restricted to the husband or partner known longest, thereby ignoring exposure to other uncircumcised partners. These investigators discovered that a considerable number of women did not know the circumcision status of their husbands. An attempt to check the accuracy of reported circumcision status by means of physical examination revealed that many men were either incorrect or uncertain as to their own status, a finding not uncommon in this type of research.[50,52-54]

Penile hygiene seems as or more important in determining cervical cancer rates than does circumcision. The interrelationship between hygiene and socioeconomic class is apparent, and high rates of cervical cancer seen in people with little education and low income may be partly a result of this factor. In a study of the environmental history of a number of cervical cancer patients and controls, Wynder[37] concludes that differences in incidence of the disease among different populations are dependent upon two factors closely related to social class: age at first coitus and penile hygiene.

As an alternative to the hypothesis that smegma acts as a carcinogen, Pratt-Thomas *et al.*[50] have suggested that something in spermatozoa could initiate cervical cancer; similarly, Rotkin[39] speculates that an agent is transmitted from the penis during coitus. Obstructive contraception, found by Aitken-Swan and Baird and others mentioned above to be used more by controls than patients, would serve to protect the cervix from these possible carcinogens.[41] Contraceptives that obstruct the cervix would also reduce the likelihood of contamination by any carcinogen transmitted by the male.

FUNCTIONAL IMPACT

In 1967 more than 23,000 women died in the United States from malignant neoplasia of the genital organs[55] (Table 9). Almost 57 percent of those deaths were due to a neoplasm of the uterus, and over one half of these uterine cancers were cervical in origin. Mortality rates from cervical cancer have fallen from 16.6 per 100,000 in

TABLE 9   Death and Death Rates (per 100,000 Population) from Malignant Neoplasms of the Female Genital Organs, United States, 1967

	No. Deaths	Rate	Percent[a] Total Mortality	Percent[b] Mortality Uterus
Malignant neoplasm of uterus				
cervix uteri	7,411	7.3	32.1	56.4
corpus uteri	1,743	1.7	7.5	13.3
uterus unspecified	3,989	3.9	17.2	30.3
subtotal	13,143	12.9	56.8	100.0
Malignant neoplasm of ovary, fallopian tube, and broad ligament	9,168	9.1	39.7	
Other unspecified female genital organs	805	0.8	3.5	
TOTAL	23,116	22.8	100.0	

[a]Based on total of 23,116 deaths.
[b]Based on total of 13,143 deaths.
Source: National Center for Health Statistics.[55]

1941–1943[11] to 7.3[55] in 1967 and continue to decline with a rate of 6.9[56] per 100,000 as reported for 1968.

Although the number of cases of *in situ* cervical cancer has increased markedly during the past 20 years, there has been little change in the absolute number of cases of invasive cervical carcinoma.[57] However, in comparison to other cancers of the female reproductive system, invasive cervical cancer appears at a younger age;[57] thus, only 4.4 percent of women with cancer of the uterine corpus are discovered before age 40, while almost 20 percent of those with cervical cancer are diagnosed before age 40.

Survival rates for patients with invasive cervical cancer increased from 1940 through 1964,[57] but have remained relatively unchanged since. Survival is related to the stage of the disease and as Figure 3 demonstrates, there has been little change among patients with regional spread of disease since 1950–1954. Whereas the 3-year survival rate for localized invasive cervical cancer is 85 percent (1960–1964), the survival rate for regional disease for the same time period is 52 percent. The 5- and 10-year survival rates for localized disease are 79 percent (1955–1959) and 68 percent (1950–1954), respectively.

Although it is obvious that cervical cancer results in significant physical and/or psychological disability, these factors are very difficult to measure. It is also difficult to quantify the economic cost associated with such morbidity. In an effort to generate such quantitative data, the Department of Health, Education, and Welfare carried out a cost-benefit study of uterine cancer.[58] Despite the many assumptions (some of which are based on tenuous data) that go into generating such estimates, these calculations do provide a provocative perspective from which to view the impact of cervical cancer. It was estimated that in 1970, 7,826 deaths would occur due to cervical cancer, with a total earnings loss of $318,754,000. Estimates were also made of the number of cases of carcinoma *in situ* that a screening program could detect and the number that appropriate teatment would prevent from developing into invasive carcinoma. Based on screening and treatment cost estimates and time lost from work resulting from disability or death, net dollar benefits of massive screening programs were derived. These calculations indicate that treatment of these cases at an early stage results in estimated net savings of over $60 million.

Although the data relating to the effects of screening are subject to criticism, the yearly total earnings loss does dramatize the women-days lost as a result of this malignant neoplasm.

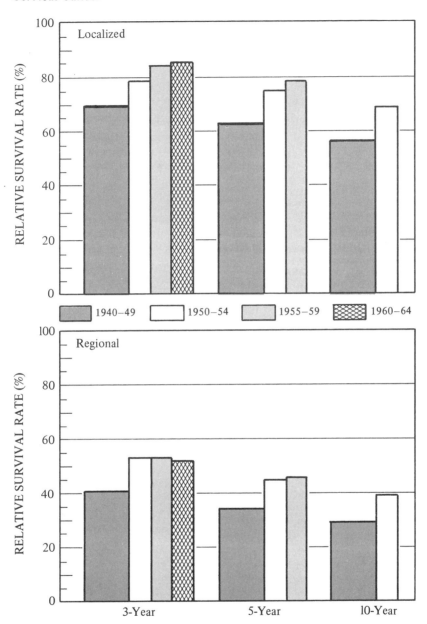

FIGURE 3 Uterine cervix: 3-year, 5-year, and 10-year relative survival rates, by stage of disease and calender period of diagnosis. From United States Department of Health, Education, and Welfare.[57]

REFERENCES

1. Doll R: The geographical distribution of cancer. Br J Cancer 23: 1–8, 1969
2. Christopherson WM: The geographic distribution of cervix cancer and its possible implications. J Irish Med Assoc 61:1–3, 1968
3. Dorn HG, Cutler S: Morbidity from Cancer in the United States. Department of Health, Education, and Welfare. Washington, DC, Government Printing Office, 1959. (PHS Publication No 590, Monograph 56)
4. Haenszel W, Marcus SC, Zimmerer EG, et al: Cancer Morbidity in Urban and Rural Iowa. Department of Health, Education, and Welfare. Washington, DC, Government Printing Office, 1956 (PHS Publication No 4621, Monograph 37)
5. Dunn JE: Preliminary findings of the Memphis-Shelby County uterine cancer study, and their interpretation. Am J Public Health 48:861–873, 1958
6. Porter JE, Stocks JF, Betts A: Incidence trends in cancer of the uterus. Trans New Engl J Obstet Gynecol 21:39–49, 1967
7. American Cancer Society: 1970 Cancer Facts and Figures. An annual report presenting the latest facts and figures relating to cancer. New York, American Cancer Society, 1970
8. Ackerman LV, del Regato JA: Cancer Diagnosis, Treatment and Prognosis. St Louis, The CV Mosby Co, 1970
9. Dunn JE, Slate TA, Merritt JW, et al: Finding for uterine cancer from one or more cytologic examinations of 33,750 women. J Natl Cancer Inst 23:507–528, 1959
10. Lundin FE, Christopherson WM, Mendez WM, et al: Morbidity from cervical cancer: Effects of cervical cytology and socioeconomic status. J Natl Cancer Inst 35:1015–1025, 1965
11. Stamler J, Fields C, Andelman SL: Epidemiology of cancer of the cervix; I. The dimensions of the problem: Mortality and morbidity from cancer of the cervix. Am J Public Health 57:791–802, 1967
12. Haenszel W, Hillhouse M: Uterine cancer morbidity in New York City and its relation to the pattern of regional variation within the United States. J Natl Cancer Inst 22:1157–1181, 1959
13. Jones ET, MacDonald J, Breslow L: A study of epidemiologic factors in carcinoma of the uterine cervix. Am J Obstet Gynecol 76:1–10, 1958
14. Dunn JE, Rowan JC, Erickson CC, et al: Uterine cancer morbidity data. Public Health Rep 69:269–274, 1954
15. Graham JB, Sotto LSJ, Paloucek FP: Carcinoma of the Cervix. Philadelphia, WB Saunders Co, 1962
16. Breslow L, Hochstim J: Sociocultural aspects of cervical cytology in Alameda County, California. Public Health Rep 79:107–112, 1964
17. Dunham LJ: Cancer of the uterine cervix in Negro women in New York City. Acta Unio Intern Contra Cancrum 17:910, 1961
18. Christopherson WM, Mendez WM, Ahuja E, et al: Cervix cancer control in Louisville, Kentucky. Cancer 26:29–38, 1970
19. Braithwaite J, cited in Kenneway EL: The racial and social incidence of cancer of the uterus. Br J Cancer 2:178–212, 1948
20. Lundin FE, Erickson CC, Sprunt DH: Socioeconomic Distribution of Cervi-

cal Cancer. Department of Health, Education, and Welfare. Washington, DC, Government Printing Office, 1964 (PHS Publication No 1209, Monograph 73)

21. Hochman AE, Ratzkowski E, Schrieber H: Incidence of carcinoma of the cervix in Jewish women in Israel. Br J Cancer 9:358–364, 1955

22. Jordon SW, Munsick RA, Stone RS: Carcinoma of the cervix in American Indian women. Cancer 23:1227–1232, 1969

23. Salisbury CG, Howard FH, Bassford PS, et al: A cancer detection survey of carcinoma of the lung and female pelvis among Navajos on the Navajo Indian Reservation. Surg Gynecol Obstet 108:257–266, 1959

24. Cross HE, Kennel EE: Cancer of the cervix in an Amish population. Cancer 21:102–108, 1968

25. Wynder EL, Cornfield J, Schroff PD, et al: A study of environmental factors in carcinoma of the cervix. Am J Obstet Gynecol 68:1016–1052, 1954

26. Martin CE: Marital and coital factors in cervical cancer. Am J Public Health 57:803–814, 1967

27. Gagon F: Contribution to the study of the etiology and prevention of cancer of the cervix of the uterus. Am J Obstet Gynecol 60:516:522, 1950

28. Taylor RS, Carroll BE, Lloyd JW: Mortality among women in 3 catholic religious orders with special reference to cancer. Cancer 12:1207–1225, 1959

29. Clemmesen J, Nielson A: The social distribution of cancer in Copenhagen, 1943–47. Br J Cancer 5:159–171, 1951

30. Stocks P: Cancer of the uterine cervix and social conditions. Br J Cancer 9:487–494, 1955

31. Rojel J: Uterine Cancer and Syphilis. Copenhagen, Nord Forlag Arnold Busck, 1953

32. Cohart EM: Socioeconomic distribution of cancer of the female sex organs in New Haven. Cancer 8:34–41, 1955

33. Lombard HL, Potter EA: Environmental factors in the etiology of cancer. Acta Unio Intern Contra Cancrum 6:1325–1333, 1950

34. Boyd JT, Doll R: A study of the etiology of carcinoma of the cervix uteri. Br J Cancer 18:419–434, 1964

35. Terris M, Oalmann MC: Carcinoma of the cervix—An epidemiologic study. Clin Sci 174:1847–1851, 1960

36. Naquib SM, Lundin FE, Davis HJ: Relation of various epidemiologic factors to cervical cancer as determined by a screening program. J Obstet Gynecol 28:451–459, 1966

37. Wynder EL: Circumcision as a preventive factor against cancer of the cervix. Natl Cancer Conf Proc 3:603–607, 1956

38. Terris M, Wilson F, Smith H, et al: The relationship of coitus to carcinoma of the cervix. Am J Public Health 57:840–847, 1967

39. Rotkin ID: Adolescent coitus and cervical cancer: Associations of related events with increased risk. Cancer Res 27:603–617, 1967

40. Rotkin ID, King RW: Environmental variables related to cervical cancer. Am J Obstet Gynecol 83:720–727, 1962

41. Aitken-Swan J, Baird D: Cancer of the uterine cervix in Aberdeenshire. Aetiological aspects. Br J Cancer 20:642–658, 1966

42. Moghissi KS, Mack HC, Porzak JP: Epidemiology of cervical cancer—study of a prison population. Am J Obstet Gynecol 100:607–614, 1968

43. Dunham LJ, Thomas LB, Edgcomb JH, et al: Some environmental factors and the development of uterine cancer in Israel and New York City. Acta Unio Internal Contra Cancrum 16:1689–1692, 1960

44. Towne JE: Carcinoma of the cervix in nulliparous and celibate women. Am J Obstet Gynecol 69:606–613, 1955

45. Harnett WL: A statistical report on 955 cases of cancer of the cervix uteri and 321 cases of cancer of the corpus uteri. Br J Cancer 3:432–473, 1949

46. Logan WPD: Marriage and childbearing in relation to cancer of the breast and uterus. Lancet 264:1199–1201, 1953

47. Macklin MT: Etiological factors in carcinoma of the uterus, especially the cervix. J Int College Surg 21:365–378, 1954

48. Levin ML, Kress LC, Goldstein H: Syphilis and cancer. NY J Med 42:1737–1744, 1942

49. Rotkin ID: Sexual characteristics of a cervical cancer population. Am J Public Health 57:815–829, 1967

50. Pratt-Thomas HR, Heins HC, Latham E, et al: The carcinogenic effect of human smegma. Cancer 9:671–680, 1956

51. Dunn JE Jr, Buell P: Association of cervical cancer with circumcision of sexual partner. J Natl Cancer Inst 22:749–763, 1959

52. Lilienfeld AM, Graham S: Validity of determining circumcision status by questionnaire as related to epidemiological studies of cancer of the cervix. J Natl Cancer Inst 22:749–764, 1959

53. Wynder EL, Licklider SD: The question of circumcision. Cancer 13: 442–445, 1960

54. Aitken-Swan J, Baird D: Circumcision and cancer of the cervix. Br J Cancer 19:217–227, 1965

55. National Center for Health Statistics: Vital statistics of the United States 1967. Volume II—Mortality part A. Department of Health, Education, and Welfare. Washington, DC, Government Printing Office, 1969

56. National Center for Health Statistics: Vital statistics of the United States 1968. Mortality. Department of Health, Education, and Welfare. Washington, DC, Goverment Printing Office (in press)

57. United States Department of Health, Education, and Welare, National Institutes of Health: End results in cancer. Prepared for End Results Group by End Results Section. Washington, DC, National Cancer Institute, 1968 (Report No 3) Government Printing Office

58. Program Analysis: Disease control programs: Cancer. Department of Health, Education, and Welfare, Office of Assistant Secretary for Program Coordination, Washington, DC, Goverment Printing Office, 1966

BIBLIOGRAPHY

Conference on Early Cervical Neoplasia, September 11–13, 1968. Obstet Gynecol Survey 24, Part 2. Cherry Hill, New Jersey, American Cancer Society, Inc., 1969

Davis HJ, Jones HW: Population screening for cancer of the cervix with irrigation smears. Am J Obstet Gynecol 96:605–618, 1966

Nelson JH, Hall JE: Detection, diagnostic evaluation, and treatment of dysplasia and early carcinoma of the cervix. Cancer J Clin 20:150–163, 1970

World Health Organization: Early Detection of Cancer. Report of a WHO Expert Committee. Geneva, World Health Organization 1969 (World Health Organization Technical Report Series 422)